LOVE IN A COLD CLIMATE

AIDS: Some Pastoral and Theological Perspectives

Edited by John Hervé

Published by CLA on behalf of the
Social Concerns Committee of the Church Union

Designed and Printed by Bocardo Press Ltd., Cowley, Oxford, England.

CONTENTS

INTRODUCTION

"Aids is the most important Public Health problem of the century, if not since the Middle Ages — Dr John Gallwey"

The implications of this are profound, both for Churches speaking out as institutions and individual pastoral practitioners caring for those for whom they are responsible. But in order to speak responsibly and care effectively, church leaders and pastoral practitioners must understand as much as possible about the nature of the problem. This is difficult as the situation changes and evolves rapidly as more information becomes available.

In response to this need, the Extension Studies Unit of St Stephen's House Oxford — an Anglican Theological College in the Catholic tradition — co-ordinated a day conference on Aids and Pastoral Care. It was inter-denominational and included anyone with an interest in the pastoral care of AIDS patients, ranging from doctors, teachers and clergy to churchwardens with a sensitivity to the pastoral needs of their congregations. The content was found to be so valuable by the participants that, following repeated requests, the transcripts appear here in printed form (with slight modifications). This material has been supplemented with a variety of other relevant articles, both sacred and secular, of a pastoral and theological nature which have a bearing on this particular pastoral task.

Thus the material follows the inter-disciplinary approach to pastoral care. John Gallwey begins, with setting out the medical facts, supplemented by the epidemiology of AIDS. This is followed by Brian Parry and Barrie Newton on pastoral issues directly related to the problem. Then there follows an edited transcript of the plenary session which, in the dynamic of dialogue, highlights many of the hitherto hidden pastoral issues. The dialogue format has been retained. These elements, apart from the epidemiology section (see acknowledgements) were the substance of the conference.

There is a growing library of material developing around the AIDS issue, of varying quality (both in accuracy and usefulness for the pastoral practitioner). So a careful selection has been made which it is hoped will help to enlarge the awareness and knowledge of all involved either directly in the care of AIDS patients or in grappling with the theological issues involved. May I commend it you as a useful addition to the AIDS section of the bookshelf of not only every pastoral practitioner and theologian but of every "thinking" Christian!

John Hervé
St Stephen's House, Oxford.
July 1987

CONTRIBUTORS

John Hervé is Director of Extension Studies and Tutor at St Stephen's House Oxford.

John Gallwey is Consultant Physician in Genito-Urinary Medicine at The Radcliffe Infirmary, Oxford, and Adviser on Genito-Urinary Medicine to the Oxfordshire Health Authority.

Kay Wellings is Research Officer for the Family Planning Association.

Brian Parry is Rural Dean of Handsworth and Vicar of St John's Perry Barr (Diocese of Birmingham).

Barrie Newton is Anglican Chaplain to St Mary's Hospital Paddington.

Jeffrey Weeks is Visiting Research Fellow at the University of Southampton.

James Hanvey is engaged in research at Campion Hall Oxford.

Martin Linskill is Dean of Degrees and Lecturer in Ethics at St Stephen's House Oxford.

Jack Dominion is Senior Consultant Psychiatrist at The Central Middlesex Hospital.

ACKNOWLEDGEMENTS

I am graeful for the help given by John Gallwey, Brian Parry and Barrie Newton in editing the transcripts of the conference. Also, Marxism To-day and Jeffrey Weeks for permission to reproduce The Epidemiology of AIDS and Love in a Cold Climate which first appeared in their issue of January 1987. AIDS and ARC: A Theological Reflection on The Church's Ministry is included by permission of The Month and James Hanvey, and When a friend has AIDS by permission of James Hanvey and St Pauls Publications. The Tablet kindly gave permission for the inclusion of AIDS and Morality which first appeared in their issue of January 1987 and The Terence Higgins Trust kindly assented to the reproduction of their pamphlet Is it Safe? — The Chalice and AIDS. Finally, the Resource List is reproduced by kind permission of The Central Board of Finance of the Church of England from *AIDS Some Guidelines on Pastoral Care* (Church House publishing 1986).

CHAPTER ONE

THE MEDICAL FACTS

Dr John Gallwey

1 WHY WE HAVE A PROBLEM

Firstly, you are all human beings. You all have a right and a duty to know about this particular problem. Secondly, you are going to be looking after people who are going to be affected by this problem. When I say affected by this problem, *everyone* is going to be affected by this problem. Some people are going to be ill. Everybody, but everybody is going to be affected by it.

Everybody is going to know someone who is ill — is going to work with someone who is ill; is going to have a patient, a parishioner, a friend or relative who has AIDS or the infection. It is important for you as people to know about this disease, it is important for you in your pastoral care to know about this and to cope with people who have problems.

In my lifetime there have been 3 great revolutions in the field of sexually transmitted diseases. The First came with the advent of anti-biotics. These lead to an amazing reduction in the amount of sexually transmitted disease; from 12,000 cases a year in Oxford in 1938 to 300 in 1950. The second revolution came with the sexual revolution of the "swinging sixties"; the change in sexual behaviour (it wasn't that people were having more sexual contact but there was more likelihood of partner change). In addition we had the development of easy communication, transport and travel. It became commonplace for disease to travel from one end of the world to another overnight. Also we had the gradual emancipation of male homosexuality in western society. There is no doubt that homosexuality is a very "successful" variation of sexuality. There are many variations of sexuality but probably the only two which are satisfying and successful are homosexuality and heterosexuality. On the other hand it carries for us as Genito-Urinary physicians some problems.

Gay men in the past have tended to have more sexual partners than their heterosexual equivalents. Some gay men have been, by any standards, bizarrly promiscuous, having many contacts; people have numbered their lifetime contacts in the thousands. That inevitably leads to the possibility of the spread of infection.

The third great revolution has come in the last 5, 6, 7 years with the appearance of a number of viral infections which are potentially fatal. The first of these was Hepatitis B, then we recognised the human papilloma virus (connected with cancer) in the neck of the womb in women, and it is worth noting that in Oxford alone 1,500 new women were diagnosed as having been infected by that virus in the past year. Then there was AIDS.

2 THE EMERGENCE OF AIDS

AIDS has presented us with major medical problems and enormous ethical ones. It first appeared in June 1981 when in the USA a number of men were identified as developing opportunistic infections and tumours. These were in people whose body defences had been severely damaged. This happens quite commonly — we deliberately suppress the immunity of people in order to transplant organs, bone marrow etc. These were people who had not had damage done deliberately to their defences for medical reasons — Gay men from urban backgrounds, and they had had a great many sexual partners. They had records and evidence of many infections, and to begin with it was thought that their immune systems were being damaged by repeated infection to the point where their immune systems were being "burnt out". This side of the Atlantic it became a popular hypothesis. We could look at the USA to say — it's your problem — it won't happen here. But it became clear that this was not correct. There were other cases among intra-venous drug users, haemophiliacs, those who had received blood transfusions, children who were born into families of "at risk" groups and sexual contacts of those in "at risk" groups. In addition, other people were seen with illnesses short of these severe, life-threatening opportunistic infections and cancers. People with swollen glands, loss of weight and night sweats. It was clear that we were dealing with a spectrum of disease caused by a blood-borne infective agent. It was actually identified in 1983/4 as a virus we now call the Human Immuno-deficiency Virus (HIV).

It used to live under many names, including the one used in this country — The Human T-cell Lymphotrophic Virus number 3 (HTLV 3). I am glad to say that tongue twisting name went and it is now known as HIV (Human Immuno-deficiency Virus). Identifying this virus allowed us to design a blood test which would help to identify those people who had been infected — the test is known as HIV anti-body test. We all know what anti-bodies are. They are protective elements which appear in the blood after infection and protect a person from further damage or infection. This is not such an anti-body! This anti-body is not able to protect — it has a little protective element but not sufficient, so don't assume that if someone has anti-bodies they are protected against damage because this is not so. We found, as you might expect, that all the people who had AIDS had this anti-body. The people with swollen glands, severe fevers,

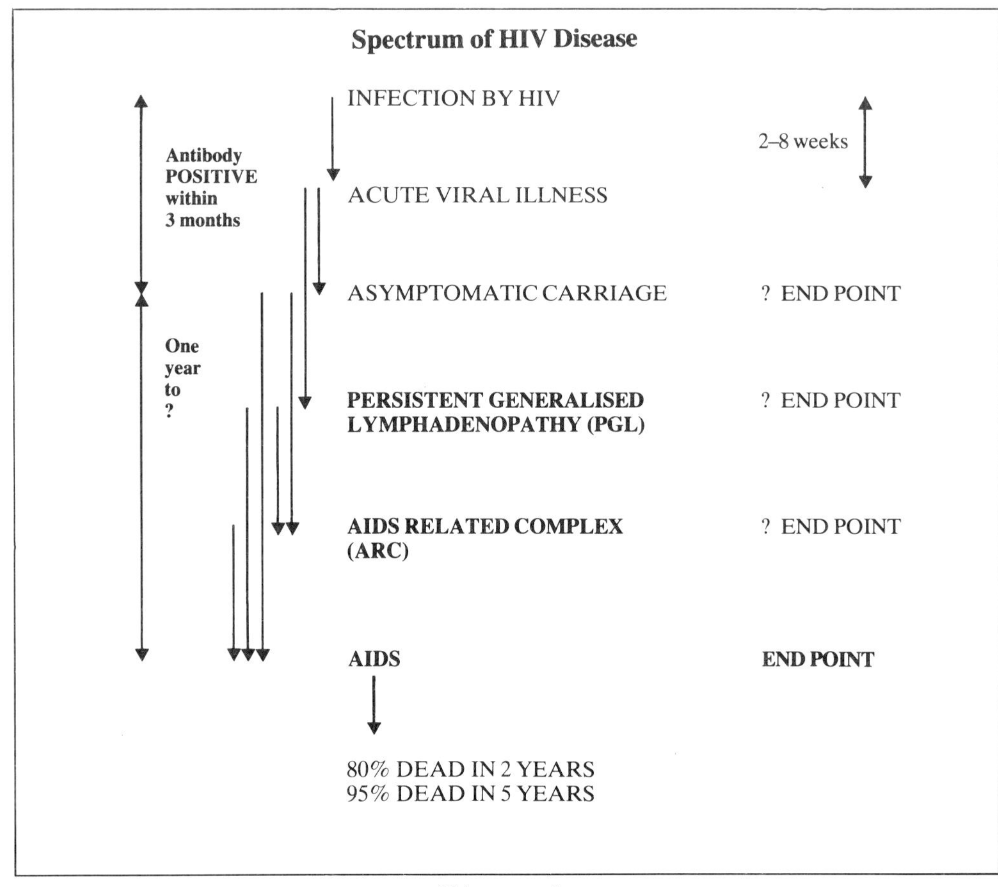

Diagram 1

severe to moderate ill-health, also had the anti-body and were infected. We call those conditions "AIDS related conditions" or "AIDS related complex". What was less expected though we ought to have logically seen it, were the vast number of people who carried evidence of infection by the virus but showed no sign of infection. They were, as we now know, "asymptomatic carriers" of the virus, because the other thing learnt about all these groups was that if somebody was anti-body positive they were carrying that virus and potentially infectious.

That is the reason why this is such a particular epidemiological problem. The Great Plague, the black death, caused major problems, but people got the infection, they died or recovered. They ceased to be infectious. With this infection, people are infected, remain infected and infectious probably for the rest of their lives. They may (or may not) get ill-health, they may (or may not) die, but it takes a long time for the full-blown syndrome to develop and therefore those people, who are unidentifiable, — except for this blood test — are a potential source of infection.

3 WHAT HAPPENS UPON INFECTION?

It is important that we all understand the spectrum of the disease and I am therefore going to expose you to medical facts which are not necessarily easy to understand. What happens is that our client becomes infected by the virus. (*See diagram 1.*) He will probably develop an acute "viral infection", rather like glandular fever. This may last a few days, it may last as long as a month or 6 weeks. He may be mildly ill and think that he has got 'flu. Or he may be severely ill and diagnosed by his GP as having a viral infection such as glandular fever. He will get over this with no problem at all (though he might be quite ill during his period); but he will make a recovery and by the end of 3 months he will be well and have developed the anti-body. The incubation period for HIV is up to and not greater than 3 months. We must be sure that when we are talking about incubation period we are talking about the time from infection to the development of the marker that tells us that person is infected.

All of these people to begin with will become asymptomatic carriers; infected and infectious. Is this in itself an "end-point"? (*See diagram 1.*) Can people spend the rest of their lives as asymptomatic carriers, having no further problems and not having their lives in any way shortened or altered by the infection? We do not know at the moment but it seems increasingly unlikely. Some people develop, very early indeed, swollen glands (what is called persistent, generalised lymphadenopathy. (*See diagram 1.*) These glands may be very obvious, not just easy to feel but you can actually see them sometimes. We have a number of patients who have several large glands in the back of the neck which can be seen quite easily. Is that an end point?

Is that compatible with a normal span of life? We don't know. What we do know is that if the glands ever disappear the person very probably will go on and develop AIDS.

Some people develop "constitutional illness". This may be in two forms. AIDS Related Complex — see diagram 1 — (moderate to severe ill health associated with fever, night-sweats, swollen glands, loss of weight, general feeling of illness, profound fatigue); it can be so severe that the person is confined to bed or is in hospital. It may be so mild that the person merely feels "one degree under", "under par" the whole time. People who develop AIDS Related Complex are likely to have remissions — that is, they will get better and then they will have another attack of the malaise. Some of them get better and return to the asymptomatic carrier stage. There was one patient we admitted and was in hospital for about 6 weeks, we really feared for his life. We couldn't prove that he had AIDS but he was clearly very ill. He has recovered; that was a year ago and he has been perfectly well ever since.

Some people develop AIDS. (*See diagram 1.*) It does such severe damage to the immune system that the body can no longer protect itself against perfectly ordinary infections. Infections such as Thrush (a common infection of the Vagina in women) — there are few women who will not get Thrush at some time or another and yet in AIDS patients this could spread throughout the whole body; it will be found in the Brain, in bone marrow, in every tissue and organ. It is treatable but untreated it would cause death. Similarly with mild infections like Herpes. In the AIDS patient, untreated it will spread and lead to death.

People can go directly from being asymptomatic to developing the severe opportunistic infections we call AIDS. This is the most shattering experience for health workers, and those who have pastoral care. The event which had the greatest effect upon the Staff of my Department was the 35 year old, very handsome, bi-sexual man who came in because he wanted to find out if he was infected. I saw him the second time he came in because he had been found to be anti-body positive. He was a good deal healthier looking than anyone else in the Department (including most of the staff!). On examination I found he had a thrush infection in his mouth, and on questioning he admitted that running up the steps to the Department he was short of breath. We X-rayed his chest and found he had pneumocystis pneumonia — the classical pneumonia associated with AIDS. We admitted him to hospital, treated him, and he was discharged after 10 days; he was very well indeed! Unfortunately he had a brain infection by then which gradually worsened and he died in a demented state after about 3 months. That had a profound effect on our Department. He was the first AIDS patient we had "seen all the way through". We were all prepared for the people who came in and began to be ill, whom we knew to be infected, and we watched AIDS develop. We were not prepared for this shattering experience. AIDS is an "end point".

People whose immune system is so severely damaged that they develop the life-threatening opportunistic infections *will* almost certainly die. After 2 years, only 20% will be alive, and after 5 years, 5%. What usually happens to the AIDS patient is that they will get an infection and it will be treated successfully. They will continue in a state of comparative health (many of them will go back to work). They will get another infection or develop an opportunistic cancer. They will be treated, make a recovery, and then they will have a series of these episodes which get closer and closer together and more and more severe. They will eventually succumb as a result of either severe infection which is untreatable, or untreatable cancer, or just sheer debility.

So, summing up, we have asymptomatic carriers which are infected and infectious. People with swollen glands, without other symptoms, again infected and infectious. We have those with constitutional illness who have developed AIDS. This presents either as infections, cancers or infections of the brain. It is becoming clearer as time goes on that many people who survive AIDS will develop brain infection and slowly develop dementia. No treatment exists for the virus and the control of the infectious consequences of immune deficiency is the best treatment strategy we have available and it will obtain for patients a better quality of life and probably a longer life expectancy. The one thing we can guarantee patients is in (and out) of hospital they will be provided with good care and that we will ensure that they do not suffer physical pain as a result of their disease.

4 DOES INFECTION MEAN AIDS?

What we want to know is the percentage of people who are infected who will go on to develop AIDS. We can only guess. AIDS has brought with it a band of people called "AIDS experts". They don't exist — there are no AIDS experts. You will find "experts" being quoted about predictions.

But we do not know! The problem has been recorded since 1981, so we only have 5 to 6 years of knowledge. We know now that by 5 years, 10.2% of people infected by the virus (however they become infected) will develop AIDS. We, however, have evidence of people being infected long before 1981 (we would have to have as the first cases were reported in that year); we know people were infected in 1975 — we have specimens of their blood which we have tested (specimens kept in storage for various research projects). We believe now that by 7–8 years, 30–35% of people will develop AIDS. An additional 30% will develop AIDS related complex. (*See diagram 2.*) In other words, illnesses short of the life-threatening opportunistic infections and tumours as AIDS. In

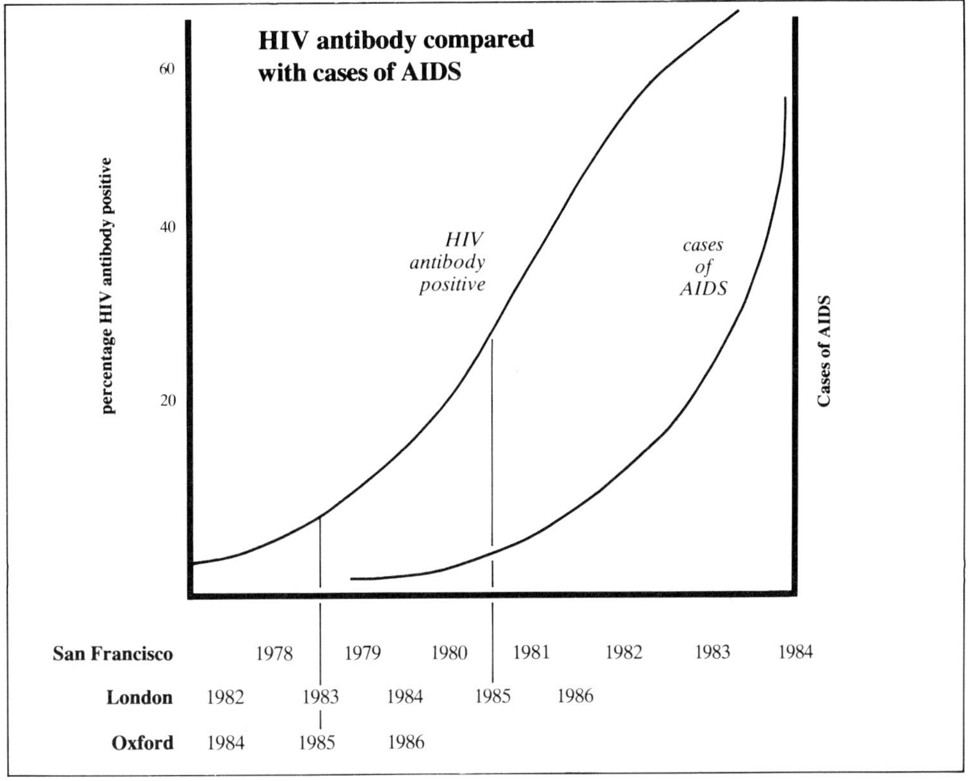

Diagram 2

addition an increasing proportion of people are developing dementia.

Now it is reasonable to say that there is no logical, biological reason why everyone who is infected by the virus should go on to develop AIDS in some shape or form. Infection, cancer, dementia — with time. Whether that is going to happen, nobody knows, so watch the "stop press". I am not going to guess if it is going to be 50%, 75% or 100%.

So if somebody is identified as being anti-body positive, what can you say about them? You can say they are infected by the virus. They are infectious and likely to remain so for life. They are not infectious every day, but you cannot say when they are infectious without very complicated and difficult investigations. They have at least a 30% chance of developing this unpleasant, lingering, painful and disgraceful disease (that is not what I am saying that it is — that is what people think it is) that they will die from in 2–3 years. They will have another 30% chance of developing ill-health which will interfere with their lives — prevent them working, going to school etc. In addition, therefore, they have at least a 1% chance per annum of developing AIDS or dementia.

That is very heavy information, and I wonder how many people here, if they think about it, could cope with that information! I couldn't. I would not dream of having the test done, nor of taking risks which might infect anyone else. But I wouldn't have the test done as I know I couldn't cope with that information.

What is the size of the problem? In the USA 2–3 million people are infected by the virus. By 1991, 270,000 will have developed AIDS in the USA and 170,000 will be dead. In 1991, 74,000 will develop AIDS in that year. There will be 54,000 deaths in that year and 29,000 other admissions to hospital. The total world cases in 1991 will be between half a million and one million. The situation in Africa is unknown. It may be that in some parts of Africa 5% of the population (Central Africa that is) are infected. These are the lucky areas. The unlucky areas may have levels of infection as high as 50%. In Uganda, in a series of blood-donors who were tested 50% had the infection. That blood was actually used — it had to be used. In the UK in the last year, 32 people a month have been infected with AIDS. 750 people have been diagnosed as having AIDS so far since we began to record it in 1981 and 450 are dead.

Put that in the context of 30,000 a year dying from cancer of the lung. But it is a different situation, because of the continued risk of infection it is an epidemic of enormous public health importance. The most important public health problem of the century, if not since the Middle Ages. By the end of 1991 we can expect 400 people a month to develop AIDS. That's a Jumbo-jet load of people falling out of the sky every month! I have no doubt your reaction is that we must do something about it. There is nothing you can do. Those 400 people are probably already infected, for if the incubation period for AIDS is around 5 years or more those people will already be infected. What we *can* do something about is the number of cases which occur in 1992, 1993, 1994 etc. The length of time from infection to developing AIDS is a number of years — it is not likely to be less than 12 months and the longest incubation period is the longest period we have known about AIDS.

5 HOW IS IT PASSED ON?

This is, I suppose the crux of the matter. This is a very fragile virus. The one thing one can say is that it is very difficult to acquire it; you have to work quite hard to acquire the infection! The virus has been identified in many body fluids and secretions. These include blood, semen, saliva, tears, breast-milk, cervical secretions, urine and the fluid around the brain (cerebro-spinal fluid). It may well be in other secretions. It isn't in sweat. It is however only important in blood, semen, and secretions from the neck of the womb (cervical secretions) the secretions that appear in the vagina. It is not going to be passed on by any other secretions.

This is quite important and not well understood. In the government's information campaign, which might be better termed "mis-information" campaign (that's rather unfair — I have the greatest admiration for any Government which has taken the steps this one has to try and curtail this epidemic) I do think they could have given the information in a different way. The exhibition of violence and phallic symbolism is extraordinary. What is immensely important is that people should not only know how the infection is passed on but how it is *not* passed on!

I suppose of all these secretions, saliva is the one people find most difficult to come to terms with. The infection is not passed on by saliva. It is as simple as that. The trouble is, it is difficult to prove a negative. People say it *could* be; whether it *will* be doesn't matter. For example, this room *could* fall in on us, but it does not. I see few people leaving the room as a result of this anxiety. The situation is the same. If there were someone I "fancied", I would not for a moment think of not kissing them because they were anti-body positive. There might be other reasons why I should think about not kissing them but acquiring infection would not be one of them! However, let me make it quite clear that if I wanted sexual intercourse with them I would not because that is the way I would acquire the infection. That is the mode of transmission.

But how is it actually transmitted? In 3 ways. Blood and blood products (in the therapeutic situation by transfusion, by the use of factors from the blood in treating haemophiliacs). 50% of haemophiliacs in this country have been infected by the use of blood products which have been infected. This will not happen any longer because we now test all blood donors every time they give blood and out of the 3 million donations already tested, 55 were positive, 51 were in groups which we expect to be infected and 4 in non "at risk" groups. However, the Centre For Disease Surveillance and Control in London thinks the other 4 people also belong to "at risk" groups but were not telling the truth (they didn't quite put it like that — they weren't that bold). People will not become infected as the result of blood transfusion or blood products except in certain bizarre situations. It is always just a tiny possibility (though it is so minimal it can be ignored). The second means of transmission is sexual contact and thirdly (sadly — all infection is sad but this especially appeals to us) the infected mother is likely to infect her unborn child during pregnancy. A woman who is infected has a 50% chance of producing an infected child and that child is likely to die within 5 to 6 years after an unpleasant and long illness.

What sort of people get infected? The main "at risk" groups — we no longer talk about "at risk" groups but "at risk" activities — are gay men and bi-sexuals, drug users, haemophiliacs and people who have blood transfusions; children of people in at risk groups; people from Central Africa and certain Caribbean Islands. They do not involve us — we can forget about it. But there is another group. Anyone with many sexual partners. We all know what a promiscuous person is, it is a person who has more sexual partners than we do ourselves. "Many" sexual partners (if I said you need to have a 100 partners to acquire this infection that would be nonsense — you only need one). Your chances of coming across somebody is larger if you have 100 sexual partners a year, as a number of my heterosexual patients certainly do. At the moment it probably *is* about 100 partners a year to turn it from *if* you get it to *when* you get it. But I don't know if it is going to be 50, 12, 6, 3 or 2! "Many" sexual partners is having *any* risk contact at all.

So what *are* the risks? Let me say that casual or accidental transmission at home, play or work doesn't happen. There is a considerable amount of evidence that supports this. No one has acquired the infection by accidental contact. You don't get it from the lavatory, from a glass, from sharing a towel, from living in the same room, from sleeping in the same bed, kissing, touching, standing next to them on the bus or underground, sitting next to someone who is infected. Think of anything and you don't get it that way! Health Care Workers are not at risk — 4 Health Care workers have been infected by accident. These were bizarre accidents where each of them injected a significant amount of blood deep into tissue — just like a drug user. The 2,000 odd Health Care Workers who accidentally inoculated themselves with a scalpel, splashing material from someone who is infected on an open wound, none of these people have become infected.

We now get on to sexual transmission which is the main way this is transmitted (apart from intravenous drug users). Sexual contact is an efficient means of exchanging bodily fluids and secretions. The only sexual activities which have been identified with transmission of the virus in the heterosexual situation are vaginal and anal intercourse. The latter is a significant manifestation of sexual behaviour among heterosexual people. We also recommend that ejaculation in the mouth is also risky. It has never been proved to be passed on this way but on first principles it is sensible not to do that. Provided a person avoids unprotected vaginal or anal contact in the heterosexual situation they will not become infected. In the homosexual situation, the only activities which have been associated with infection are penetrative anal intercourse. We know it is easier for a man to infect a woman than a woman a man. It is easier for the insertive anal partner in a gay situation to pass on the infection than for the receptive anal partner. In other words, vaginal intercourse is a riskier situation for a woman and receptive anal intercourse is riskier for a gay man!

6 HOW CAN PEOPLE PROTECT THEMSELVES?

So how can people protect themselves? There is no doubt that in an exclusive pair-bond relationship, whatever type of relationship it is, gay or "straight", where neither partner is infected, there is no risk in any sexual practice. There is no doubt, then, that the greatest protection is monogamy. Our belief is few people expect to have a single sexual partner in their life-time. Indeed, would that be a good thing? If people reject monogamy, then the use of a condom is a protection. It does not give absolute protection (let me remind you of that spurious statistic that if a couple got married and had intercourse 3 to 4 times a week until she was menopausal — and they used a condom on every occasion — they would have a family of 6 children!). So it is not a perfect protection against conception or pregnancy and is not a perfect protection against infection. But it is a good deal better than nothing.

So we promote the use of condoms. It is second best to monogamy, serial monogamy, and if people are trying to obtain serial monogamy we would suggest that they avoid intercourse until their relationship is established (or if they do not avoid it that they use a condom). That is our message. That is the Government's message. We are dealing with a condition, problem, epidemic which is easier to prevent than an epidemic of influenza. By a change in behaviour, stopping people using drugs and everyone using a condom, the epidemic would stop at that point. But we are dealing with behaviour which is difficult to change, and the people who are least accepting our message at the moment are those who *most* need to change their behaviour — young heterosexual adults who are changing partners. The homosexual community, in the vast majority, have changed their behaviour; our levels of infection in homosexuals living in Oxford is virtually nil — from one of our greatest problems it has become one of our nil problems.

7 WILL THERE BE A VACCINE?

Control depends on vaccines — we have no vaccines. They are difficult to produce and it is unlikely that we shall have them for a number of years. Drugs? Perhaps there will never be a curative drug. This is simply because this is a virus that so incorporates itself in the human body that we would need a whole new concept of medicine; an ability to cut a piece out of individual cells without actually affecting that cell. It seems unlikely that would ever exist. Palliative drugs — these are given to someone infected and can reduce ill-health and morbidity. They already exist but unfortunately at the moment are unavailable in this country (AZT is one of them). They have considerable side effects so are only given in the "life threatening situation". We can screen people to see if they are infectious. It has value (and should be mandatory) in the donor situation where people are donating blood, organs, semen or tissue. It could be voluntary in, for instance, pregnancy and in an area where there is a high risk of infection. We next voluntarily test the "bridging groups" — those groups of people who can carry the infection from the "high risk" groups to the general population. We can offer it to people in "at risk" groups (homosexuals or heterosexuals).

8 SO WHAT NOW?

At the end of the day, what we have to concentrate on is education, behavioural modification and morality. There are a number of people "climbing on the bandwagon" of AIDS in order to make their bigotry respectable or force people into their morality. That is not, itself, moral behaviour. Fear is not a useful way of promoting responsible attitudes. Yes, fear and practicality do come into this; moral values will probably change for the human race could be brought to a halt — it may be brought to a permanent halt if we don't solve this problem! We need public awareness. We need people to understand how it is caught and how it is *not* caught. Above all we need people to have compassion for those at risk, compassion and understanding for those infected. We need to give care to those people who are ill. Now we are coming to pastoral care which is *your job!*

CHAPTER TWO

THE EPIDEMIOLOGY OF AIDS

Kaye Wellings

One of the most striking features, epidemiologically, of the AIDS epidemic, has been the cliff-face rise in the numbers affected. Since the first recorded case of AIDS in the UK in December 1981, the figures have doubled every eight to 10 months to reach 512 in September this year. In the US the rise has been even more dramatic.

The exponential growth rate of AIDS (a steady rise in the rate of increase as well as in the actual numbers) has prompted some wild statistical speculation as to how high the figures might go. Simply projecting the current rate of increase into the future would give an estimate of nearly a million cases in Britain by the mid-1990s.

But these kinds of predictions assume that the disease will spread as rapidly in the general population as it has in high risk groups, and that people will not change their behaviour significantly. Most epidemiologists are of the

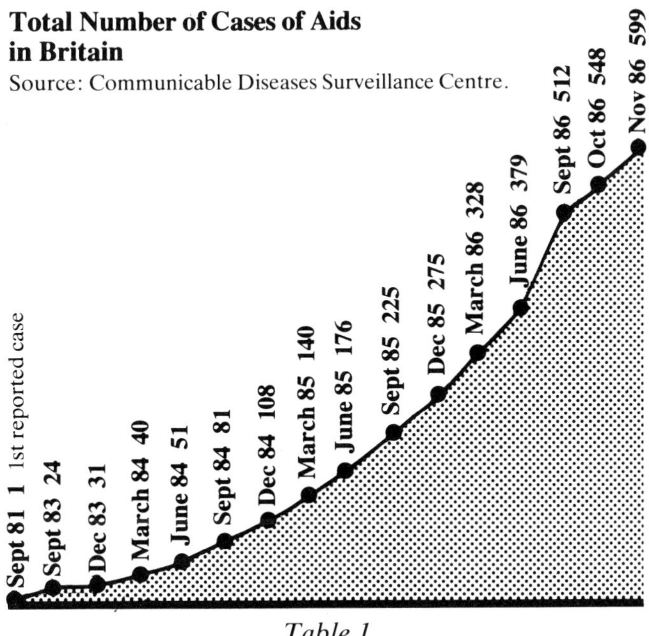

Table 1

Reported Cases: Europe and North America

Country	Total to June 86
USA	24,491
Canada	699
Switzerland	138
Denmark	93
Belgium	171
France	859
Netherlands	146
Iceland	2
West Germany	538
Luxembourg	3
Sweden	57
UK	389
Norway	24
Italy	300
Austria	36
Spain	17

Country	Rate per 100,000 of population
USA	10.5
Canada	2.8
Switzerland	2.12
Denmark	1.82
Belgium	1.73
France	1.56
Netherlands	1.01
Iceland	1.00
West Germany	0.88
Luxembourg	0.75
Sweden	0.69
UK	0.69
Norway	0.57
Italy	0.52
Austria	0.48
Spain	0.46

Source: Hansard Nov 4, 86

Table 2

view that AIDS will plateau out as a steady state is reached.

Even so, the rise in numbers is likely to continue for the foreseeable future. Around 30,000 are thought to be infected with the virus in Britain, an estimate seen as conservative by some. The US figure for the total number of cases, which was roughly the same five years ago as Britain's is now, stands today at more than 25,000. (For international comparison see Table 2).

The spread of the AIDS virus has moved beyond the risk groups originally identified as the four Hs (homosexuals, heroin addicts, haemophiliacs and Haitians). Official figures in the West have, admittedly, provided some grounds for seeing the disease as affecting mainly gay men. In Britain, for example, they account for nine out of 10 recorded cases and in America seven out of 10.

But there has always been ample evidence from further afield that AIDS is just as much a heterosexual disease. In parts of Africa, Zaire for example, the ratio of men to women sufferers is 11 to 10, and cases do not fall into the recognised risk groups.

The African connection helps explain varying rates around Europe. Higher than average rates in Belgium and France are no doubt in part due to the larger proportions of Africans in the population.

CHAPTER THREE

CARE OF AIDS SUFFERERS

a personal experience – Brian Parry

I shall begin with a quotation from a Christian Counsellor with AIDS patients in the USA. "Dying with AIDS is horrible, living with AIDS is dreadful."

The probability of anyone here having to care for an Aids sufferer at home, is thank goodness fairly remote for the present, but we do not know what the future holds for anyone in the caring professions. Perhaps my own experience was unique in this country in that three years ago to this time of the year, I began to care for an AIDS sufferer in my home.

What I feel I must establish first of all is that it is perfectly possible to undertake such a caring role in the home environment and what any agency involved with this disease needs to do is to promote and support all efforts for sufferers to be able to live what lives they have left in the comfort, happiness and stability of a normal home life.

The second thing to establish is that there is no cause to fear such a possibility, it seems that those who have been involved in research into the virus are now certain that it cannot be passed on in normal social contact. With normal hygiene and direction from professional medical people there is NO risk to the carers. There is in fact a much higher risk with other diseases which can also be fatal.

Obviously it will not be possible to care for some patients outside the hospital situation and as with Peter, periods in hospital care will probably be necessary because of treatment for some of the opportunistic diseases which develop. Nevertheless from my own experience it was possible for Peter to spend long periods at home and achieve a great deal during periods of reasonable health — the most important thing was that he was able to die at home.

I feel I must stress that there are physical demands of the carer so it is essential that you keep healthy yourself and realise that you may need outside help. I shall always be grateful for the necessary assistance I had from friends both of Peter and myself, the people of my congregation and of course the doctors and nurses both inside and outside of hospital.

Care is not all for a sufferers physical needs, in fact the pastoral care from both the spiritual and mental aspect is equally important. Obviously I can only speak from my own experience. The pattern of needs will obviously differ but I can't help feeling that the basic needs will be similar for the non-Christian or Christian. I will consider the personality needs as I call them as opposed to physical needs in the order that Peter seemed to experience them.

The first was Fear in the form of panic which became heightened as soon as the diagnosis was confirmed. The sort of questions he asked are: What is going to happen to me? Will it be painful? How long have I got to live? Will I be able to get proper treatment? No one can possibly have all the answers to such questions so it is important to establish from the outset that the carer may need support and professional help from doctors and counsellors to equip them for the role they are in. I think that this could be particularly so with a non-religious person because of the absence of hope for a future and better life.

One important fact which I do want to stress is that the carer needs to have as much information as possible concerning the illness, its implications, what can be done to keep the sufferer as healthy as possible, you do in fact become a life line to the person. Again it is essential to lead as normal life as possible in the home, sudden changes from routine could cause panic and make the person feel insecure remember we are dealing with Fear/ Panic and for this condition there is no better antidote than knowledge of the situation and security.

The second experience was Shame. For a long time to come there will be a stigma attached to the disease. If the person is gay they will be aware that homosexuals are being blamed for the spread of the disease. It can in many instances be the means, unintentionally, of "Coming Out" and involve very difficult situations between family and friends. We must take into consideration that unless the illness has been contracted through blood or blood products a very intimate area of one's life is made public and lets face it sex is still a very naughty thing in many areas of society so the carers may find themselves being the informant to family and friends of sufferers. I can't think of anything significant I did to help Peter deal with his intense feelings of shame except to encourage his family and friends to love and support him and to point out that he is still the same Peter who they had known and loved before discovering he had AIDS.

The third experience is closely associated with the shame. There will obviously be rejection from some people but this is also an experience within the person even if they do not come directly into contact with such people, they could be aware that rejection is a distinct possibility. So there will be a need to rebuild confidence from time to time, physical illness does weaken our confidence in normal circumstances. You cannot rebuild such confidence alone it will be important to involve relations and friends who still love and care and you may also be responsible for educating them about the "ins and outs" of AIDS, in order to give them confidence. BUT and this is a big BUT, don't overwhelm the person with visitors or helpers because I am absolutely certain that the sick person will need a lot of space and time to work out their own solutions to feelings and problems and they will frequently feel very physically ill. What will be more constructive than lots of casual visitors will be the genuine love and acceptance and reliability of a few real relations and friends who are aware that they need to relieve the feelings of rejection and also be an example to those who may have rejected the person.

Fourthly, I want to return to Fear, not so much the panic kind of fear experienced when the illness is confirmed, but the fear of the inevitable unknown (death). This again I feel could be a little easier when caring for a committed Christian. Peter eventually wanted to die, his body was absolutely finished and he had arrived at a stage when he had complete faith and trust in God and was at peace with all who mattered in his life and above all with himself. I feel that this is something which a carer should try to encourage in a sufferer whether they are Christian or not. Although we had been friends for ten years and Peter had made his home with me for eight years apart from two periods when he branched out on his own, I was still his parish priest and was therefore able to exercise an extra area of caring but remember if any of you undertake such a responsibility, you will have to care for and minister to someone who is dying. There were moments of intense fear particularly when there were serious declines in his health and strength. I recall one particular instance when I had to take him into hospital in the middle of the night, he was so scared I couldn't even leave him to go to the loo after waiting for admission for at least two and a half hours. I could do little for him physically on many occasions but just being there, holding his hand, embracing him, did I know help at such moments. Each sick person will have different needs, each carer will have different skills and methods, the most important thing is if you care then get in and do it, to help give someone something valuable in their lives even in these circumstances is rewarding and I do believe that every human being has the right to die with dignity and surrounded by those who love you.

I found myself with grief, physically very tired and alone with difficult thoughts of how unjust it was that a vital and caring young man should be cut down by a disease he didn't deserve. And then who cares for the carers? Fortunately there were many who did care for me, this could be your role, perhaps not as intense and involved as caring for an AIDS patient but I think equally as important.

Finally we must also be aware of those people who know that they are anti-body positive. We do not know yet what the prognosis is for those who carry the virus so all of them are living with fear and may have to drastically alter their life styles, they too need support and care and at the moment these are much more numerous than those people who actually have AIDS.

CHAPTER FOUR

AIDS – THE PASTORAL IMPLICATIONS

Barrie Newton

I am not an "expert" — I am a Chaplain to a General Hospital which happens to have acquired quite a large share of responsibility for caring for people with AIDS and infections associated with it. Though I do spend a large amount of my time in the Isolation Unit I do have responsibilities elsewhere. Also, it is not only the Chaplains who are giving pastoral care. Sometimes I have to queue to see patients as there are so many people waiting to give pastoral care! Being in London, we have charitable support from the Terence Higgins Trust, Body Positive etc. We have some excellent Social Workers specialising in the pastoral care of AIDS patients and Clinical Psychologists (who are not nearly as frightening as that title sounds). My pastoral care is only a small part of what patients receive — but a very specialised part.

I have always felt that the Church, through both its ministers and members, has a great deal to say to those who are ill and a great deal more to say to those who are dying. My experience in relation to AIDS is limited to one hospital, and in this context the patients we tend to have at St Mary's are gay men — we do have others but the majority fall into that particular category. This is partly due to the fact that for many years we have had an enormous Sexually Transmitted Disease Clinic which has been quite well thought of in the gay community for having been non-judgmental, "anonymity preserved if required" etc; so gay men with STDs come to St Mary's Hospital, and when some of them develop AIDS they stay with the Hospital and the Doctors they had come to know.

What I would like to do is tell you of some of the problems I have come across in the Hospital and hope that you may see parallels in your own sphere of work — whether it be Hospital, Parish, School, or College.

I realised from the outset that the Church had a lot of "leeway" to make up. Soon after I got to St Mary's I was seeing a patient who was very welcoming and friendly. After I had seen him a couple of times he said "You are the Hospital Chaplain aren't you?" I said "Yes". He said "I am surprised you will even talk to me, let alone be sympathetic!" That reaction was produced by his reading of the newspaper where "a Churchman" said "If my son said he had AIDS I would shoot him!" (and "a Churchman" was often being quoted in the paper at that time denouncing people who got this "disgusting illness!"). For this patient to find someone wearing a dog-collar who could bear to be in the same room was quite an eye-opener. So in many areas we still have that problem, though thank goodness the churches P.R. on the subject is a bit better now!

So I realised that first of all I had to establish myself as a human being. A lot of this is no different from the pastoral care of anyone else. The Pastor needs to establish him/herself as a fellow human being who can try and understand and share. The patients at Mary's are nursed in single wards — this has been forced upon us as we use an isolation ward. We don't have an "AIDS Ward". There are people in that ward with all sorts of other things as well (which helps when you are trying to preserve confidentiality). It does not follow at Mary's that if you are in "Ward X" you have AIDS.

The problem in hospitals which have a ward specifically for nursing AIDS sufferers is that it is impossible to keep the diagnosis confidential. We have single rooms, doors with glass panels and a "flap" so you can peer in and see if the patient is free. Our staff approve of this as it gives the patient privacy; also, having this illness gives rise to times of deep emotion both for the patients and those who love them. Privacy is necessary so that these emotions can be expressed and so that those involved can "cry their eyes out" if they want to (without the nurse having to draw curtains around). But single rooms can also isolate the patients. This is one of the reasons why they are often pleased to see the Chaplain — someone who is coming in to talk and break down the isolation. That may be why I have had a generally friendly reception so far! I always knock on the door; I always say "I am the Hospital Chaplain, may I come in?" If they say "No", or "I'm tired" or as one man said "I want to finish reading my paper", I go and see someone else. They have an absolute right to say "no thank you" and patients in hospital should always have that right to refuse visitors of any kind. I usually spend the first visit establishing general points of contact or mutual interest to establish myself as a human being — and not some kind of "weird being". This is because the reputation of the Church, particularly on the subject of homosexuality, is not good and a number of the men who come into Mary's will, because of their past life-styles, have a low opinion of the Church and clergy. I think this "low impression" is thoroughly deserved on our part and I can't help feeling that gay monogamy would be much more widespread if the Church did not make it so difficult for people to form gay relationships! If it hadn't been necessary to keep quiet about your "special friend" you might not have gone up to London to find lots of "special friends" one after another. The disapproval you would have brought upon yourself because you had tried to live with a person of the same sex might also have been the cause of moving away to find, in the first place, some privacy. If we hadn't imposed that kind of judgmental attitude on people maybe there would have been more settled relationships and less need to "sleep around" (and therefore perhaps, less of the illness around). I think we have to own up to our share of responsibility for the state of the gay culture in this country in certain respects.

Having said that, when patients find that the Chaplain is an ordinary person, its amazing how much, and how profoundly, they will talk. Some of them are practising church members of various kinds. Some will want the same sort of pastoral support in hospital anyone of this background would want; they want the sacraments, to go to chapel, to be prayed with and blessed. Can I lay to rest a myth and underline what Dr Gallwey said: we have a chapel at Mary's and everyone is welcome. We celebrate the Eucharist there twice a week and patients receive the sacraments in both kinds. At no stage has any of our doctors said that we should not administer the chalice in the Hospital Chapel. I am quite sure that if there was any risk at all, the Hospital Chapel would have been the first place where advice would have been given to stop. Despite all the conflicting letters in the Church press last week (some from Doctors I see) you will have some reassurance from Dr Gallwey and myself — and by implication from our Doctors at Mary's that there is no risk at all. Some of you may know that the Anglican Bishop of California when he is celebrating Mass always receives the sacraments last — I don't mean he just consumes what is left — he makes a point of administering the chalice to everyone else in the Church before it touches his own lips. That's one kind of gesture to show people not to be afraid. Please help people not to be afraid!

So there is the ordinary pastoral support. We had one man — a brilliant University Lecturer — in whom the illness eventually took the form of affecting his brain and virtually "scrambled" it. He couldn't see or talk coherently — he could just about hear. All he wanted to do was have the Bible read to him. So my Lay-Reader colleague and I used to take it in turns to visit him. First of all we would read the passages of the Bible he especially liked and asked for; then when he was no longer able to ask we would use the passages we thought he might find comforting. I blessed the name of the Gideons at that time for the lists they put into the front of the hospital Bibles of "which part to read when you are . . . . ." — it was a great help! One was able to give — even when he was beyond receiving the communion — the Sacrament of the Word of God.

One man had asked, when he knew he was at the end of his life, for the Sacrament of the Sick. That was a very fraught situation. I was told the man had a sister who had stood at the end of the bed and denounced him a "notorious evil-liver" which wasn't a great help to him (or anyone else). She had to be quietly removed from the room. I heard about this, and when he asked to be anointed I went up to the ward. I hoped some of the family would be there — I always think it is more meaningful to have some of the family or other people there with you — and there were some people in the waiting room. I went in, met them briefly, and said how much I admired John's courage and the dignity with which he was approaching the end of his life. I noticed a slightly "tight-lipped" look on the face of the woman and it turned out she was the one who had been "blasting-off" at him just before-hand! I don't know if my opinion did anything towards changing hers but she came into the room. I explained to the patient what I was going to do — he was still compos mentis enough to understand. I also invited one of the nurses in (it is no news to those working in hospitals to know how encouraged and strengthened the patients are to have a nurse with them when they are receiving the sacraments). She was finding it all a bit much, but she stood near the door in the background. Having explained to John what I was going to do, I said "Now before we have the anointing, let us pause and think of anything in particular we want to ask God's forgiveness for" and after a pause we said the Kyries — Lord have mercy, Christ have mercy, Lord have mercy.

The thing that affected us all deeply was that all through the rest of the service John was saying "Lord have mercy on me" very quietly — which was appropriate and desperately moving. It was one of those occasions when I was glad I know the words off by heart because I couldn't see the pages of the prayer book! Everyone was like this — the brother-in-law, nephew, and the poor nurse by the door. As soon as we got to "Amen" she was out of the door and gone! By the time I joined her in the rest-room she was half way through a cigarette. She could see my eyes were "fuzzy" too — we sat in the rest-room and made a cup of instant coffee; put our arms around each other, reached for another NHS Kleenex, blew noses, mopped eyes and went out to face the world.

The strain on the staff is a heavy area of pastoral concern in hospitals. There is very great emotional stess and strain on people caring for AIDS patients and one of the roles of the Priest (as Hospital Chaplain or Parish Priest) is supporting church members who are Doctors and Nurses. I drink interminable cups of coffee with them, listen to how awful it is for them; and I get my sixpennyworth in telling them how awful it is for me. We sympathise with each other, have a rest, a break, or arrange to go out for a drink or something in the evening. Then we shrug our shoulders and get on with it the next day. But it isn't easy. They've tried Staff Support Groups (but these haven't worked) not because people didn't want them but they haven't time to go to them!

The pressure on beds in London hospitals at the moment is enormous and at Mary's it is exceptionally heavy because we have closed one hospital and not opened our new wing yet. Here is one brief example: in the ward there is a "white-board" on which the bed number and name of the patient is written on it. I went in to check who was in which room the other day and it said "Room 10, James and Chris". Now I thought I know they are very broad-minded on this ward but (a) I didn't think we had any double beds and (b) I wasn't quite sure what the nursing authorities would think about this. I found to my horror that one chap was in for a couple of days and the other was only in for tests in the day time. So the one in for a couple of days went and sat in the day-room and the man in for a few hours used the bed and then went home. It gets very difficult and there is stress in sorting out who can come in and who can't.

All of these things pile up onto the Doctors and nurses, so as well as the difficult decisions as professionals, they also have extra decisions about who should be treated with the limited resources available and this all helps to weigh them down. Having said that, there is also a great amount of joy to be found on our isolation ward. Joy at seeing just how human beings can care for each other (I don't mean only the people who are paid to be there, I mean the families, partners, lovers, and so on). On that Isolation Ward on the fifth floor there is more love per square foot than in many places (more, I must say, than in many Christian congregations). There is a unity of purpose; total acceptance of the patient as a person; no hint of criticism or denunciation or "second-class-citizen" approach from anybody. That is apart from the odd one or two who break in (and soon get short shrift). One (non-Anglican) Clergyman was discovered standing at the end of a bed saying "Repent of your evil ways". He was thrown out by the sister, luckily via the door and not the window! He is an exception — it's a very loving place to work and when the church is seen to be loving as well it is interesting how the "un-churched" or non-Christian on the staff notice. When you have a family totally "in the picture" surrounding the patient with love, presence and prayers, the agnostic and the unconnected notice. They think perhaps Christianity is not as awful as they thought it was. They get caught up in this love and Christians and non-Christians alike are united in caring for people in need. It is a very encouraging and marvellous place to work for that reason.

One of the biggest problems is the secrecy with which many of the patients have surrounded their private lives in the past. Many are from outside London and come into it because the atmosphere is freer and easier. They could have friendships with people of the same sex, settle down and live together more easily, so life in London is totally divorced from life at home. There will be parents and relations who haven't the faintest idea (a) that the person is gay and (b) they have an illness only "those funny people get" anyway! One of the pastor's problems is helping patients decide how best they can cope with their own families. And we have had two particular total disasters in that area. One was a young man whose parents had not the faintest idea that he was gay, and he had caring for him someone who had been a lover and was by then just a friend — but a very devoted friend. The friend knew what was happening but the parents didn't. I doubt if you can imagine any situation so fraught as going into a room in which all the three people are — two not knowing and one knowing totally — and trying to give pastoral support to that "mixed bag".

When I am asked — which I am sometimes — my suggestion to the patient is that it is always best to be as honest as possible. On the other hand, its always best to tell as *few* people as possible. That situation was fraught because the mother knew that boys of 32 don't die of pneumonia these days; and that was what she was being told was wrong with him because he said before he was put on the Ventilator (as a result of the pneumonia) "do not tell my parents". The staff are dedicated to preserving the patients confidentiality. Much as we should have liked to have talked to him about it, suggested that there might be difficulties, and would he like to reconsider, we didn't have a chance. To the end they honoured his request and the parents weren't told. This created an enormous amount of tension between the staff and the parents, the parents and the friend, and so on.

Another similar case was a chap from Scotland whose parents lived in a little village miles away from the nearest city; they didn't know what was going on with him in London and his brother who also lived in London did a marvellous job trying to persuade parents that "he is ill, dying, he loves you, I presume you still love him — it doesn't matter". But they couldn't cope. Everytime the Doctor came in to talk to them the mother got up and walked out;"I don't want to hear this" she said. Even when the Doctor came to say good re-assuring things she couldn't cope. In the end, the parents moved out of the brother's flat in which they were staying because they couldn't accept the way he was trying to help them change the attitudes of a lifetime. They couldn't face the pain of going back to their village and people knowing that their son was "one of those homosexuals". The brother told me afterwards that everyone in the village knew! But the parents couldn't cope and we didn't manage between us to help them to cope.

It would be presumptuous of me to tell you how to be pastors, and it would be silly, because the pastoral care of "x" is different from the pastoral care of "y". One thing I would urge of you when caring for patients with this illness (whether in hospital or at home) is that you do everything to break down their feelings of isolation. The best way to do this is to put your arms around them! (Or at least hold their hand.) I spend a lot of time with my arms around people — which is comforting for me and I hope them as well! One of the best ways of caring for people who feel isolated is to hug them. As Dr Gallwey said, there is no danger from kissing people either, and the more human contact they have the less they will feel isolated from the human race generally (and despite all the loving care of Nurses, Doctors, Chaplains and others they still do feel terribly isolated). Their "cover has been blown" for many of them on their life-style which they have been trying to keep secret; their parents may have abandoned them (though I must say that for those I have met so far this hasn't been a problem). The problem has actually been trying to persuade people to take turns in visiting so that the patients don't get too tired!

Being abandoned by lovers and partners hasn't happened much at "Mary's". Being abandoned by family unfortunately has. It may well be that working in parishes its the pastoral care of the parents, brothers and sisters and children which may be a bigger problem for many of you. The basic rules are still the same. One of the things about talking on this subject is that it is possible to say a lot and not touch on the one thing you had hoped I was going to say. So I will stop talking and try and "field" any questions; or please, those of you who have experience of pastoral care of those with AIDS share your experience if you would like to.

Question — Is the confidentiality for AIDS victims continued even after death? I am dealing with a mother who is half convinced her son died of AIDS though the death certificate didn't say it. Nobody said it to her at the time of death. She was unsure yet frightened to go to the doctor and ask. Is confidentiality a handicap in pastoral care in this situation?

Response —
BN: It is true as far as I know that no death certificate has AIDS written on it. As you know, anyone can go to the modern equivalent of Somerset House and look up a death certificate. Unfortunately, with greater education newspaper reporters can identify the AIDS infections; if these appear on a death certificate they may well assume that it was a question of AIDS. The problem with the lady concerned is whether she really wants to know or not. Perhaps I might refer this to Dr Gallwey. As you know, lots of information about people who died of AIDS has got into the papers after death. I assume confidentiality continues after death (but) people have ways of breaking it. I don't think anyone has the right to demand details of diagnosis.

JG: That is correct. Confidentiality beyond the grave — one has to use ones common sense and humanity. There may be the situation where she doesn't want to know. It may be the situation where it would be more valuable for her to know. This is a situation which should be discussed along a spectrum of people. It may be that the clinician himself is not the best person to choose, it may be the sister on the ward, the Chaplain, the representative of the Terence Higgins Trust. One has to be careful about confidentiality. If I might just tell you about one particular case and the disaster in this instance. The son of a Clergyman who returned to his country home unwell was admitted to hospital. He was found to have AIDS. He knew his family could not cope with his information — he wanted it withheld. One of the nurses on the ward told the mother we think we know what it is, it is a type of pneumonia. The mother was so pleased — she had a diagnosis — she went home and told the whole village. She was the only person in the village who didn't know what the diagnosis meant. So we had the situation of the family not knowing but everyone else in the village knowing. As a result of that the Doctor rang me and asked "could you ask this chap not to come to church for Holy Communion but to arrange to have it at home? — I said that the Bishop of Oxford had said there was no risk, but you have to realise the parishioners in this church are not just ordinary people, they are retired Bank Managers, Stock-Brokers and people like this. I said that no, I would not have suggested this. The doctor replied that in that case he knows half the parishioners would go elsewhere. This is the sort of problem which can arise.

BN: Has the mother, as Next-of-Kin, the right to ask for the diagnosis?

JG: She has the right to ask; I don't know if she has the right necessarily to get the answer! Confidentiality must go beyond the grave, but personally if I think it would be valuable, and if others like yourself think it would be valuable, then it is reasonable to tell her. That's what would happen in Oxford. What would happen at St Mary's I don't know.

BN: Is that any help?

Questioner: Yes, I suspect the son actually said "whatever you do, don't tell Mum". This has been respected and is actually quite detrimental to her.

BN: It might be that it needs to be "re-negotiated" in some way. You have pastoral care of this lady?

Questioner: Unfortunately no. He was in the forces and so I have no contact with the medical authorities concerned.

Question — Would you comment further about Staff Support Groups?

BN: Staff Support Groups are alright, but if you are going to have them then you have to have other staff who are going to look after the patients whilst staff attend the groups — and those we haven't got! I don't know about groups outside the hospital. I think that outside the "work area" support comes from individuals (neighbours, Womens Institute, whatever). I can't see any way we could organise a support group outside the hospital. Everything comes down to the shortage of staff. If we had more nurses we would be able to relieve pressure on them and give them breaks and time to talk this thing over.

Question — Following the recently publicised views of the Roman Catholic hierarchy, do you find Roman Catholics turn to you for support?

BN: No. RC patients in S Mary's do talk to me and I visit them quite a lot. Several of them still practise their religion and go down to communion. We did have a patient from QUEST (the RC equivalent of the Gay Christian Movement) who was critical of the hierarchy but still went to Mass (which is quite right and proper!).

One last thing. Doctor Gallwey talked about this room falling down; the word AIDS has been said in this room several times and it hasn't collapsed. I suggest that if you said AIDS in your church occasionally it wouldn't collapse either. In the intercessions, remember people who have AIDS; when using prayers for hospitals remember Dr Gallwey and his staff; and make it clear that you don't have to wash your mouth out with carbolic after you have said the word in Church — and that will be a start!

CHAPTER FIVE

PLENARY SESSION

The title of the groups indicates the special area of interest around which discussion centred. In the dialogue occurring in the plenary session, abbreviations are as follows:

SP: Spokesperson
JG: Dr John Gallwey
BN: Fr Barrie Newton
BP: Fr Brian Parry
Comment: Comment from the floor

1 MEDICAL GROUP

SP: Our discussion was quite general. One thing we did talk about was the care of AIDS patients who were dying and about hospice provision. We decided that it would probably be better if there were not special hospices, for these further the social isolation of AIDS patients. Wherever possible, people should be able to die at home with adequate support.

JG: I agree on both points. The difficulty is that many hospices at the moment are saying that within their terms of reference they are not allowed to take AIDS patients — I hope this will be resolved over time. If it *is* necessary in the course of time to found specific AIDS hospices, many in the medical profession feel it would be better to add a small space onto existing hospice premises. It is important that we do not establish "leper colonies". The second point made by the group is also valid. All patients, whatever their situation, have the right to die at home. Perhaps Barrie would like to comment?

BN: Hospices exist to keep people out of them until it is absolutely necessary. Our hospital has a policy that patients should be cared for at home as long as possible. It is unfortunate that at the moment, some London areas have no policy on home care. Others such as Camden, Kensington, Brent and so on have established home care teams. In those areas where they are not provided, people unable to get out for their shopping, to cook their meals, etc, have to be admitted to hospital. There are plans for a hostel near the hospital which will give people temporary housing in between hospital visits and there are plans for the "London Lighthouse" which is going to be a major AIDS centre including hospice beds. We need money for home care teams.

JG: In the USA they have found a "half-way-house" useful; that is, sheltered accommodation for AIDS sufferers. Whether these come into being here depends on the whole community — influencing legislators and health authorities to provide these facilities. The voices of caring people need to be heard.

SP: Another thing we talked about was the information given to the population as a whole. People are not accustomed to reading what appear to be specialised leaflets and ways could be evolved in which leaflets are discussed informally in groups and speakers from statutory and voluntary organisations could give information and questions could be asked.

BN: If the leaflet was more straightforward in the first place then this would not be necessary. The DHSS (1987) leaflet tried hard but didn't quite make it. The Terence Higgins Trust leaflet does "raise the blood pressure" of some sections of the community, but at least it uses day-to-day vocabulary.

BP: There must surely be a continuing programme of general education. A leaflet going into peoples homes or a short informative series on television is not sufficient.

JG: At the moment we are engaged in a priming exercise. The generations which are still at school and which are not yet sexually active should be given a wide knowledge of the situation and there should therefore undoubtedly be changes in sexual behaviour because of this. But this priming exercise is a most difficult and important one.

SP: A final point we made was that counsellors should, when engaged in face-to-face encounters and using phone-lines, use explicit and clear language.

2 EDUCATION AND YOUNG PEOPLE

SP: Our group was looking at what is going on in schools — or more accurately, what is *not* going on in schools. We thought that information was not being given to young people at primary and secondary levels of education. One of our group is Head of a primary school who said some people may think that primary levels of education are not relevant to such a discussion; but areas of discussion with such children must cover all aspects of their social, personal and health education. This is vital, otherwise the myths attached to AIDS (eg. it is the "gay plague") will continue.

JG: It may seem inappropriate to children in primary schools, but they can read, they watch TV and will hear and know about AIDS. It is a matter of "tailoring" information to be appropriate to that group. I don't think that a 7 year old child who asks about the disease needs a lesson in oral sex but they can be helped by appropriate information — AIDS must not be a mystery to them like Father Christmas, i.e. to be explained to them when they are older!

Comment: Would you agree that specific people ought to be appointed for such tasks?

JG: I think the way the Oxfordshire Area has tackled it is good. Namely, the Health Education Unit has set up a team of people who will provide a series of seminars for up to 500 educationalists. During these they are exposed to knowledge of the virus and ways of exploring their own attitudes. It is hoped that at least two people from each school will be at these. Their job will be to go back and design a course appropriate to their own schools.

BP: I remember — as a child — the poster "keep death off the roads". Children remember such advertising and we need to provide accurate education around social issues.

JG: Another valid point in this regard was made by a school governor at a meeting I attended recently. It was that we must be careful not to destroy any healthy attitudes towards sexuality that children may have or should acquire.

BN: What is slightly worrying is that schools which are trying to educate in this regard are not helped by childrens' social perceptions outside the school — they watch TV for instance and see many people being promiscuous without taking any precautions etc.

Comment: I would like to endorse what Fr Newton has said. There does seem to be a generalised hypocrisy where the media is concerned for they never seem to mention contraception and yet promiscuity is often promoted as a social expectation.

3 DEATH, HOSPICES AND MORTALITY COUNSELLING

SP: Most of our group discussion is reflected in the previous ones, but there are two things we would like to highlight.

(1) Although we were undecided as to whether there ought to be specific AIDS hospices, we did think that the care of those with the disease should be dealt with in the same way as the hospice movement has developed already — namely in a pioneering spirit. That is, both in caring for AIDS patients themselves and in making the public aware of the nature of the disease.

(2) We also reiterated the point that it is easier in cities for gay people to "come out". If they live in a smaller community it is more difficult to come to terms with the fact that you have AIDS and that people are going to know that you are gay. So what does such a person do? The point was made that in every community there is a church. These could at least set up information centres (there is a great deal of literature available from organisations like the Terence Higgins Trust). So even in the smallest communities there would be somewhere for people to go for information and even practical help. The greatest fear is fear of the unknown. Churches can tell people about the nature of the disease, what happens if they have it, and give practical help and support to people with it!

JG: Clergy and religious people need to "come out" — that is, to stand up and say "we care about AIDS; we are here and we want you to come to us, let us know who you are and we will help you". You must be seen to be available.

BN: Would that every Parish church was seen to be a centre of compassion and love generally, let alone for people involved in AIDS related issues. We should constantly aim for this.

BP: Every Parish Church and Priest has a duty in this regard and we must surely work towards this aim.

Comment: We must also be aware that we have to deal with pseudo-AIDS as well, that is the condition of fear about the disease. What you might call "afrAIDS".

JG: Clergy must know about AIDS issues and gain experience in dealing with them. Many will not go to their GP — he is often seen as a "NON-confidential" person. But most people do know that a priest will never disclose anything. People are returning to using Clergy as counsellors where they have moved away from their doctors scientific approach.

BN: I would see the need as more nurses and beds in hospitals. We have the creature comforts in hospitals (thanks to Leagues of Friends, Terence Higgins Trust, etc.) but need money spent on the basics.

JG: Also, care of the carers is most important. In the USA it is thought that people can only work in the field of AIDS for about 3 years — they are "burnt out" because of the pressure of work. Counsellors in my own department (who are not necessarily dealing with those with the full AIDS syndrome but with those who think they have it or those who are infectious) are "close to the edge" because of overwork.

BP: I would like to support that. There is a whole area of care needed for those who are infected but who do not have the full AIDS syndrome.

JG: I would argue that people who are identified as being infected have *greater* anxieties and *greater* psychiatric morbidity than patients with the full blown AIDS syndrome. The other point I would like to make is that, strangely, the only group of people who have not offered their help to my Department have been Clergymen!

4 RESOURCE ALLOCATION

SP: One question was raised by the treasurer of OXAIDS who asked what the priorities of financial provision ought to be now. Phonelines or other areas? Also the point was made that AIDS is not only a problem for gay people, and yet Government advertising does not seem to be making heterosexual people stop and think. Should advertising be geared more to heterosexual people? Finally, the point was made that has featured from another group — namely that speakers from organisations such as the Terence Higgins Trust should be asked to speak to congregations etc.

JG: The priorities for spending at the moment, it seems to me, are

(1) Helplines so that they may be available 24 hours a day, 7 days a week.

(2) Training speakers for educational purposes.

(3) Counselling and support training.

5 THE RESPONSE OF THE CHURCHES

SP: One of the problems of Clergy speaking about AIDS is that we speak with a different voice. The Archbishop of York, on the one hand, says that if we are in doubt where the chalice is concerned then we should use intinction. Doctors, on the other, say that there is no danger at all. Also, the moral stance of the Church always seems negative. We wished that we had a positive ethic we could promote. We also wondered if we should preach sermons about AIDS.

We have two specific questions:

(1) to Fr Parry — Did you have any problems with people receiving the chalice at your church, knowing that someone in the congregation had AIDS?

BP: 18 months after the event, yes.

(2) to Dr Gallwey — Mention has been made of pregnant women in Scotland. Are the

mothers told if the test is positive, and if so, what advice is given (eg. is abortion recommended)?

JG: A major issue here is people's definition of promiscuity. What is it? Is it the number of partners people have? If so, what is the number? Is the person who has a number of meaningful relationships a promiscuous person? Or is it the person who has one sexual contact with a person they will never know? Promiscuity is something we need to come to terms with and to understand. The dictionary definition is "indiscriminate". That is certainly my definition. The person who has 1,000 sexual partners must be promiscuous, but not necessarily the person who has 10.

Comment: I think we must acknowledge the behaviour reflected in TV dramas for they are more influential than we might think. Monogamy is not made exciting. How do we put it across in the media that it is a possibility?

Comment: I am an RC priest and one of the difficulties I have come across is that as an RC priest I have an allegiance to my church and its moral teaching. Cardinal Hume has done a good job in such things as his article "the moral renaissance". It is interesting that on Channel Four he has said that the Catholic Church has always previously seen promiscuity as sinful — now it has become suicidal. He also said that the Government is now trying to do what the church has done for centuries, except that fear is going to prove a more effective preacher. There is a difficulty in remaining faithful to the teachings of the Church and exercising care for those who have AIDS.

JG: As probably the only agnostic in the room I feel I can challenge your comment. I find it extraordinary that church leaders can feel it useful to achieve their purpose through fear. If that is part of belief I will accept it, but surely the end can't justify the means.

Comment: I think what Christian leaders are trying to say is not that fear should change behaviour but that the gospel message is acceptable. That Christian morality is an acceptable way of life.

Comment: Isn't it the case that all churches put burdens on people? For they all condemn homosexual relationships — they do not see them as being compatible with Christianity. Dorothy L. Sayers said that it is the function of the Christian Church to bring good out of evil. AIDS has focussed the minds of many people on the condition of homosexuality; until now it has not been acknowledged that many homosexuals are Christians. Now they have to be openly ministered to. So on the one hand we are to condemn them and on the other follow the specific teachings of Christ and love and care for them. Surely the churches need to come to terms with the whole issue of sexuality in general and homosexuality in particular!

7 ETHICAL ISSUES AND COUNSELLING

SP: We discussed the problem of compassion for individuals versus the question of principles. We felt that:

(1) Counsellors need to be aware of the up-to-date facts.

(2) AIDS is not "the gay plague" or confined to homosexuals.

(3) Confidentiality of diagnosis can pose difficulties in pastoral care when exercising this for friends, relatives, etc.

(4) Specialist bereavement counselling will be necessary, especially in situations where rejection has occurred.

BP: On the point of individual compassion versus principles — we have to be careful about this in the counselling context. If you are counselling someone there is the non-judgemental element to be taken into consideration. If you are counselling a Christian who is concerned about the moral dimension, then this introduces another element to be taken into account.

JG: There are circumstances in counselling, surely, when you have to direct a person along a certain path — a path of responsibility and morality. For example, the person who is found to be "positive" and whose wife or partner is not (and he is not going to tell them). Then you may actually say to the patient that you think their action is wrong, I cannot be tolerant of that and defend your right to do that. I will respect your confidentility because you are my patient but I think what you are doing is wrong. You may alienate the patient by doing that or, more likely, they will change their behaviour.

8 PASTORAL CARE AND JUDGEMENT

SP: Most of the subjects in our workshop discussion have been raised already. One point that was made was that we have often grieved and agonised over the Church. A body which says many different things on the same ethical issues, is often judgemental, missing many opportunities to care for people in need in this country.

BN: I would agree generally with that, but there are church communities in this country who are doing their caring and showing compassion very effectively; especially in relation to AIDS. We have not had one church member with AIDS who has not been visited regularly by members of their congregation, received the ministrations of the clergy and often visited by their Bishop. This is quite encouraging.

CHAPTER SIX

LOVE IN A COLD CLIMATE

Rarely has a disease carried such powerful moral and social overtones. At last, however, the government has been forced to act. **Jeffrey Weeks** looks at the aids crisis

Aids may be the most serious health crisis to face the world this century. But during its relatively brief history it has become more than a ghastly and relentless disease. It has come to symbolise an age where fear, prejudice and irrationality battle against reason, responsibility and collective endeavour. At the moment it is by no means clear which will triumph.

The reasons for fear are real enough. Some 10m people worldwide may be infected with the HIV virus, the cause of Aids. Many, perhaps most, of these will go on to get the full blown syndrome. In the USA there have been 25,000 cases of Aids, and 10,000 dead. It is estimated that up to 2m people carry the virus. Aids is already the major cause of premature death among adult males in many North American cities. In parts of central Africa the disease is rife. In the next five years up to 1.5m cases of the illness are expected on the whole continent.

The UK figures are less dramatic but still worrying. There are probably already more than 30,000 HIV carriers. Over 550 people have been diagnosed as having Aids. Half of these are dead. And the number of people with Aids doubles every 10 months. Cases of Aids are expected to rise six-fold by the end of 1988, to envelope 3,000 people.

This is a major worldwide health crisis. It has been likened to the great plagues that ravaged Europe in the Middle Ages; and to the influenza epidemic at the end of the first world war, which wiped out more people than all the fighting on all the fronts of the war itself.

But this health emergency seems all the more frightening because, at least in the West, we have grown accustomed to the triumphs of medicine in controlling disease. Even with this virus, medical science has shown its efficiency. We now know about HIV — *except* how to destroy it. In the meantime, the incidence of Aids doubles every 10 months.

This is the background to the British government's new sense of urgency. After months of prevarication — it apparently took a last-ditch direct appeal to the prime minister by the permanent head of the DHSS and the chief medical advisor to wrench her into action — the government has set up a cabinet-level committee to coordinate action. An unprecedented health education campaign has been launched, with press, radio and TV advertising, a leaflet drop on 23m households, and a £20m budget. The health secretary, Norman Fowler, has echoed the words of his advertising copy: 'Stick to one partner; if you don't, use a condom', And for drug misusers, 'don't inject drugs; if you can't stop, don't share equipment.'

In the absence for the foreseeable future of a cure or of a vaccine to prevent the spread of the virus, the only safeguard appears to lie with changes in people's behaviour and with the public education needed to achieve that. This has been clear for some time, and has been the burden of all the expert advice and all the pressure from the groups in the population most affected.

It is some indication of the prejudice and irrationality surrounding the disease that it has taken so long for the government to adopt a high profile policy on prevention. Here Aids ceases to be simply a devastating disease and becomes more like a battlefield for conflicting moral and political values, and ways of life.

The popular response to Aids, the fear and loathing it evokes beyond the actual impact of the disease itself, illuminates a wider crisis of norms and values. Attitudes towards Aids, and the tardy political reaction, have been shaped by the fact that from its first identification in the USA in 1981 it has been strongly associated with marginalised, oppressed or feared groups; with Haitians, and subsequently with black Americans (a disproportionate number of American victims are black); with intravenous drug abusers; and with male homosexuals.

Aids has fed easily into wider anxieties and fears that find a focus in powerful streams of racism and homophobia. The result has been predictable and disastrous: a 'moral panic' rooted in a genuine fear of the disease, but seeking scapegoats in those who were the chief sufferers from it.

Moral panics, waves of social anxiety which bring to the surface deep currents of feeling and fear, generally arise in situations of confusion and ambiguity, in periods when the boundaries between legitimate and illegitimate behaviour seem to need redefining or reclassification. There is a typical stereotyping of the main actors as peculiar types of monsters, leading to an escalating level of fear and perceived threat, the taking up of panic stations and absolutist positions, and a search for symbolic solutions to the dramatised problem.

In the case of Aids there was a real, anxiety-making disease for which there was no cure, and which seemed to be localised amongst certain groups of people. Irrationally, but predictably, the form the panic took was the search for people to blame. Normally, those suffering from a terrible illness evoke sympathy. Here the victims themselves were stigmatised. Those with Aids were easily divided into two categories: the 'innocent' (haemophiliacs, female partners of bisexual men, children), and the 'guilty' (drug addicts, the 'promiscuous' and gay men).

But it is above all the linkage of Aids with homosexuality that has dominated attitudes. Aids is not a specifically homosexual disease, let alone a 'gay plague'. In the Third World it is overwhelmingly a disease amongst heterosexuals. But in most Western countries the main incidence of the illness so far has been amongst gay men. It was only when it began to dawn on people in the past few months that Aids was a general danger that the more scabrous papers like The Sun began to talk of a world health crisis.

The response to Aids is, however, more than a moral panic. Trying to understand it is like watching a speeded-up film about the postwar world. Many of the major fears, imagined threats, genuine changes and paranoias pass rapidly before our eyes: the 'break-up' of the family, the presence of 'alien wedges', that elusive phenomenon known as 'permissiveness' . . . It is above all changes in sexual mores that have come to symbolise for many people, and especially the moral Right, all the other changes that have taken place. For the former solicitor general, Sir Ian Percival, the reasons for Aids were transparent: because 'so many have strayed so far and so often from what we are taught as normal moral behaviour'. And as in many of these debates, it is the 60s that has become the symbolic focus of these changes.

There have been three major strands in the moral and sexual shifts of the past generation: a secularisation of moral attitudes, a liberalisation of popular beliefs and behaviours, and a greater readiness to value and respect social, cultural and sexual diversity. The significance of the Aids crisis is that it can be used to call into question each of these, and to advance a justification for a return to that 'normal moral behaviour' which acts as a yardstick by which to measure the presumed descent into the present.

One of the major changes in the organisation of moral behaviour over the past century has been the progressive detachment of sexual norms from religious ones. By the 1960s many of the christian churches themselves, ranging from the traditionally liberal Quakers to the established Church of England, had effectively abandoned any attempt to impose their own moral values on the whole of society. A distinction was now made between individual morality and social order, with the role of the state being redefined as guaranteeing the latter, not meddling with the former. This was the position broadly endorsed in the great wave of 'permissive legislation' in the 1960s, which reformed the law on homosexuality, abortion, censorship and divorce.

These changes were never accepted by moral conservatives nor by all the churches, and since the 1960s a gathering storm of moral absolutism and social purity has developed. In the USA a combination of television evangelism, big money and religious fundamentalism joined hands with new right forces to create the moral majority ('Neither moral nor a majority'). Britain is unlikely to see the emergence of quite such a potent force, but on a range of issues from teenage sex to the representation of sexuality, a moral Right has been mobilised, stretching from the moral rearmament enthusiasms of Mrs Mary Whitehouse to the post-feminist traditionalism of Victoria Gillick, backed by a number of more sinister figures playing their tune in parliament and elsewhere.

Aids has proved a golden opportunity for these moral entrepreneurs to raise their profile, to prove to their own satisfaction at least that what they had said all along was true. In recent years there has been growing anxiety about the effects of sexually transmitted diseases such as herpes and hepatitis B. If Aids is similarly a disease that can be transmitted sexually, then it must prove that 'promiscuity' is not only wrong but, in the inimitable words of a Tory MP, it 'kills'. And gay men, traditionally described as 'promiscuous', and the main victims of the disease in the West, thus become symbolic of the whole moral decline. As Mrs Whitehouse characteristically put it: 'Over recent years homosexuality has been represented as being perfectly normal. . . But now the laughing is over.' In the age of Aids, it becomes easier to believe that the limits of medicine and of science have been reached. It therefore makes it potentially more acceptable to seek a moral explanation. 'If Aids is not an Act of God' thundered the ineffable John Junor in the Sunday Express, 'with consequences just as frightful as fire and brimstone, then just what the hell is it?'

This moral revivalism must not be exaggerated. A general liberalisation of attitudes has sunk deep roots since the 1960s, and with it has gone a new willingness to tolerate, if not fully accept, sexual diversity. There has been no major breach in the liberal legal reforms of the 1960s, despite several attempts to restrict access to abortion. Mrs Gillick's early legal victories in her efforts to pevent doctors providing contraceptive advice to girls under 16 proved phyrric. Tory MPs may yet succeed in tightening the laws on obscenity, but despite a huge Conservative majority their successes so far have been limited. Even the saloon bar moralist Peter Bruinvels has stated his opposition to attempting to make homosexuality illegal once again.

It is difficult to take Norman Tebbit's attack on the permissive society too seriously when his colleagues are caught dealing with prostitutes and having sex in public lavatories. It seems a little hypocritical to attack one parent families (which junior minister Rhodes Boyson recently did) when one of your former colleagues notoriously contributed to founding one. It must also be a trifle embarrassing to crusade against drug abusers when the children of Her Majesty's ministers are amongst them. Senior ministers are products and victims of the major cultural changes of the past generation like everyone else. It does not mean that they will not ride the whirlwind of reaction, but what they can do will be constrained or shaped by the political balance of forces rather than by pure prejudice.

There is considerable evidence that popular attitudes continue to liberalise on many issues, from pre-marital sex to abortion and divorce. There is a greater acceptance of diverse lifestyles and of varied domestic patterns. Even the stigma of illegitimacy is now set for the history books.

There are, nevertheless, significant cross-currents, and homosexuality in particular is caught up in them. Opinion polls suggest that a clear majority of the British public are now against discriminatory laws. But 52% in a recent poll would still prefer not to have a homosexual neighbour, and nearly 70%, according to the British Social Attitudes survey, refuse to recognise the legitimacy of lesbian and gay relationships.

Yet, along with the rise of feminism, the emergence of public lesbian and gay presence has been one of the most dramatic changes in the social and sexual scene over the past 30 years. From being a love that barely whispered its name it has now become highly vocal.

These changes have not gone unnoticed. In the USA mobilisation against homosexuality has been a significant element in the new Right's efforts to shape a new majority. Just as feminism can be blamed for profoundly disrupting traditional demarcations between the sexes, homosexuality has been attacked for undermining marriage and the family. Lesbian and gay ways of life are deeply antithetical to the 'pro-family' rhetoric and authoritarian moral values espoused by the new Right.

And the whole issue of the legitimacy of non-traditional sexual relations is a fraught one beyond the bounds of the new Right. Consider for instance the torment and convolutions of the Archbishop of York, Dr John Habgood, in an interview in the Daily Mail. He did not, of course, want to see homosexuals 'beleaguered, threatened and shunned by society.' On the other hand it was unwise to go to the other extreme. He confessed to regarding homosexuality as a 'misfortune', and he was opposed to seeing homosexuality and heterosexuality as 'two perfectly viable alternatives'.

For the Left it is an even more difficult topic, cutting across traditional political positions and disrupting other loyalties. The pro-gay policies of the London borough of Haringey, under a radical black leader have been bitterly opposed both by sections of the white working class and by militant elements in the black community, because of their supposed threat to the family.

There has been an 'unfinished revolution' in attitudes to sexuality in general and to homosexuality in particular. There have been many fundamental changes in the past 30 years, but their impact has been uneven and fragmented, producing frustration as well as social progress, new tensions as well as the alleviation of old injustices. Secularisation, liberalisation, changes in the pattern of relationships have all taken place. But they have left deep residues of anxiety and fear, which Aids as a social phenomenon has fed on and reaffirmed.

Aids is not a disease of a particular type of person. It has affected, and killed, heterosexuals and homosexuals, women and men, white and black, young and old, rich and poor, the promiscuous and the inexperienced. It is the result not of a way of life but of a virus. Moreover, despite the nature of the illness it causes HIV is not a particularly strong or infectious virus. This is why Aids is not transmitted through the air, nor by casual contact, nor by even quite intimate activity such as kissing. It is spread only through the exchange of bodily fluids, particularly vaginal fluids, semen and blood.

Some groups of people are currently more at risk than others. But it is misleading to talk about 'risk categories'. This inevitably leads to a confident belief that it is always someone else's disease. The identification of Aids as a 'gay plague' has potentially disastrous effects. It not only leads to the stigmatisation of the disease itself, but it also encourages those who do not see themselves as gay to believe they will not get it.

It is not high risk 'categories' that spread Aids, it is high risk activities, those which involve the interchange of bodily fluids. These include genital and anal intercourse without protection, oral sex which involves the swallowing of semen, sexual practices (like fist fucking) which might rupture delicate blood vessels, oral-genital sex, and drug-taking where needles are shared.

'Promiscuity' as such is not the danger. Obviously, the more partners you have the more likely you are to come into contact with someone who is carrying the virus. But it is not the number of partners that constitutes the real danger, it is what you do with them. Nor does drug abuse alone lead to Aids. It can only do so when blood is exchanged via dirty needles.

Given that at the moment there is no cure for Aids, and there is unlikely to be one in the next few years, what is clearly essential is that people change their habits sufficiently to avoid high risk activities. Other 'solutions' are clearly impractical or unlikely to work. Injunctions to lifelong monogamy might seem a simple solution, as might giving up drug abuse. But in practice, as the government's advertising effectively concedes, our social natures are a little more recalcitrant than that.

The moral Right has offered more draconian suggestions. These have ranged from the compulsory testing of those at risk, including everyone coming from those parts of Africa where the incidence of Aids is high, to the segregation of the infected and sick. Leaving aside the racism of these proposals, and the affront to civil liberties they represent, they would demand an unprecedented mobilisation of resources, and would still not stop the virus. Tests are sometimes unreliable; they cannot take account of subsequent infection; and there is virtually no means by which segregation of huge numbers of people could be effectively policed.

The Thatcher government has not yet ruled out compulsory testing of immigrants, and it is still conceivable that it will make a symbolic gesture along these lines to assuage pressure (opinion polls suggest that there is an overwhelming public demand for compulsory testing of the whole population). But such steps will not stop the spread of Aids.

The two practical parts of Norman Fowler's advice to the nation — to use condoms, and avoid sharing needles — are thus not only sensible, they are essential. It has, however, taken a great deal of anguish to reach this stage. When Mrs Thatcher saw the draft of the first advertising campaign in early 1986 she is reported to have vetoed them with the comment: 'it's like writings on a lavatory wall'. Beyond this are a clear range of anxieties for moral conservatives: would promotion of the use of condoms promote promiscuity? Would mention of anal sex encourage the impressionable to try it? The minutes of Lord Whitelaw's committee will make fascinating reading in 30 years' time.

Even now, certain obvious steps have been baulked at. Advertising has not stressed that free condoms can be obtained for 'family planning' purposes. Despite the support of the health ministers, the government is reluctant to offer free needles to iv drug users from fear that it would be seen to condone drug abuse. Yet something momentous is surely underway. British governments have been traditionally reluctant to intervene too directly in the details of sexual regulation. During the last war millions of condoms were distributed to soldiers as a preventive against VD, but the fiction was maintained that these were to be used to protect the barrels of guns. Here, for the first time, we see a highly conservative government urging its citizens to use protectives, in a massive programme of sex education.

Sex education has been a touch-stone issue for the moral Right throughout the West. Publicly provided sex education has been seen as a means for the undermining of parental authority, and as a channel for the promotion of sexual perversion 'on the rates'. As the Thatcher government was contemplating its leap into openness in relation to Aids, it was also wrestling with attempts by its backbenchers to remove control of sex education from teachers and a growing controversy about the 'positive images' policies of Labour-controlled education authorities. Simultaneously, the education secretary, Kenneth Baker, was pandering to pressure from his right-wing by denouncing a gay sex education book for children, Jenny Lives with Eric and Martin, whose main message seemed to be that gay men could be monogamous too. Yet now we witness the government attempting the biggest, and most radical, sex education programme of all.

The deep waters it is entering are likely to produce ever more challenging tests to the government's moral principles. It has been propelled by the potential enormity of the problem to go further in offering explicit advice than would have seemed conceivable only six months ago. It has done so because Aids has ceased to be a minority problem, or a problem of troublesome minorities. It has belatedly been recognised as a problem for the whole of society.

The only really important question we need to ask is: how will society cope?

The evidence from the gay community suggests that people can change their habits in response to a perceived danger, and a sense of their responsibilities to themselves and others. The incidence of sexually transmitted diseases has, for instance, dropped significantly — by up to 70% in some London STD clinics — suggesting the impact of sustained community-based campaign for safer sex.

Many of the support organisations like the Terrence Higgins Trust and Body Positive (for those tested positive for the HIV virus) had their origins in the gay community, and are still to a large extent sustained by it. Clearly, if the public education campaign is to work for the whole population then continuous assistance needs to be provided for help organisations such as these on a major scale. (It has been estimated by British Telecom, for instance, that following the inauguration of the government's campaign in November, the Terrence Higgins Trust was receiving 400 phone calls per minute; its resources only allowed it to deal with one).

Voluntary effort, however important, is clearly not enough. The government has bitten the bullet on public education. It still has to confront the resource implications of the fight against Aids. Labour's spokesman on health matters, Michael Meacher, has estimated that the government needs to spend up to five times the amount currently allotted by the government. Aids illustrates above all the need for preventive medicine, for a first-class health service, for collective provision. Yet it has erupted into a political situation where all these are underfunded or under sustained attack.

There are many other challenges. Insurance companies refuse protection to those they deem at risk. People with the HIV virus as well as those with full-blown Aids are finding themselves discriminated against in jobs and housing. Local neighbourhoods campaign virulently against the establishment of hospices for the dying. Children with Aids face prejudice at school. Even private hospitals, darlings of Mrs Thatcher's health policy, refuse to take Aids patients . . . The list is potentially endless.

And looming over all these domestic problems is the possibility of a catastrophe in parts of the Third World, especially Africa, where Aids is caught up in a cycle of poverty and disease that only a massive redistribution of resources from the North to the South can begin to tackle.

Aids is much more than a medical problem. It throws a bright search light into the complexities, contradictions, divisions and needs of the modern world. It poses many difficult moral and political challenges. It is still too early to say how these will be met.

On the negative side is the evidence of popular prejudice and government sloth over the past five years. On the positive side is abundant evidence of commitment, courage and responsibility: from the medical profession, from scores of volunteers and from people with HIV infection of Aids themselves. There are two systems of values at play. The future history of the Aids crisis depends on which one wins.

CHAPTER SEVEN

AIDS AND ARC: a theological reflection on the Church's ministry

James Hanvey SJ

I wish to acknowledge my indebtedness for the help and generosity of the AIDS/ARC programme in the diocese of San Francisco. The time I spent working with them was deeply enriching not least because of their own courage and compassion.

The phenomena of AIDS and ARC (AIDS Related Complex) has been taken up by the media and is increasingly in the public conscience. It is clear that the disease is unique, not only in its physical effects but also in the moral, social and political questions to which it gives rise.

At present, there are many groups who are engaged in deeply compassionate care, making their resources available and giving powerful witness to human solidarity in the face of a very destructive illness. Each one comes with a particular perspective and philosophy, but because of the fundamental nature of the issues it is perhaps of the Christian Community that AIDS/ARC asks a special question. It is not simply 'Can you help?' or 'Will you help?' There is a deeper level of interrogation: 'Who are you and what is the meaning of *your* ministry among so many others?' This question is not only present in the case of any life-threatening illness especially one fraught with such complexity, but it must be the fundamental question of every ministry if it is not simply a singular event of crises response. The individual Christian and the community are constantly called not only to act but to reflect upon the meaning of their action, if it is to remain an action open to the Spirit and one which carries the integrity of faith. Action and reflection are part of a critical and corrective dialectic through which the community seeks for apostolic authenticity.[1] A ministry which is grounded in this dynamic will be a ministry of power.

THE CONTEXT

The present estimates of those diagnosed with the disease and the future projections more than justify public attention and concern.[2] Contrary to the facts, it is still a disease associated with gays and I.V. drug users. In addition, it also touches upon two great taboo subjects of our society: death and sex. It is a disease for which there is, as yet, no cure and its long, silent, incubation period undermines the faith we have been taught to have in the omniscience of medical technology. In this climate, AIDS/ARC has not only met with the public distaste and embarrassment which have, in the past, accompanied other diseases such as cancer or polio; it has been surrounded by fear and paranoia, militating against a throughgoing assessment of the problem and the allocation of resources.

However, behind the statistics and the reports are the people themselves, their families and loved ones. There are the children who are born with AIDS[3] whose life begins under threat and the haemophiliacs who are accidentally infected. There are people from every class and level of education; those who are articulate and financially secure with supportive families and friends and those whose lives have been spent on the streets, and who are already the victims of poverty, drugs, or just inadequacy. There are those with deep resources of faith and spirituality and others who are isolated and alone whose only friend is death. Yet all are marked with a disease which places them on the margin of society or frequently confirms their place there. In the case of those who are gay, AIDS/ARC exposes them to the moral judgements and conventions of a heterosexual society. Often the illness is seen as a consequence of lifestyles which transgress against the mores of this society and are presumed to be the result of sexual promiscuity and indulgence. Even where there is compassion, because of these prevailing assumptions, there can often be a reservation in the response.

AIDS/ARC therefore, is clearly a complex phenomena, not only biologically, but in the way it exposes our values and fears as well as our political and moral defence systems. It is a disease which relentlessly places before our society the basic questions of life and death, love and fear, individual rights and needs balanced against those of the wider community. As well as being an occasion of compassion and courage, it also exposes deep seated and unexamined prejudices. It is for this reason that AIDS/ARC does not belong to any sub-group or race: it is something which questions us about the quality of our society, our humanity or the lack of it.

In *On Being a Christian* Hans Küng writes a description of Christ's first followers that could, with minor exceptions, be a description of persons with AIDS or ARC:

> This people, a flock without a shepherd, feeling misunderstood by both the establishment and the rebels, despised by the pharasaical devout individuals of the towns and villages and by the ascetics of the desert, useless for either temple or military service, incapable of exact observance of the law and still less of major ascetic achievement: this is the people on whom Jesus has compassion. . . these who are called blessed, who are not enfranchised, who can be neglected and abused with impunity at all times by the ruling parties and authorities: these must feel he understands them. They are for him. (p.279)

THE BASIS OF A CHRISTIAN MINISTRY

There has already been a vocal Christian response which says that AIDS/ARC is God's punishment.[4] Although the majority of the major Christian Churches have rejected this interpretation, it bears some examination for it raises some important questions about the theological basis of any ministry of the Church.

To assert that AIDS is God's punishment is to take the question out of the purely medical forum and place it in the theological and moral one. This is a necessary and legitimate shift: any Christian response clearly presupposes that a purely medical understanding is necessarily incomplete. However, the perception of AIDS and ARC in moral terms is worked out on the basis of a causal connection between moral failure (and/or sinfulness) and the acquisition of AIDS — AIDS becomes the just consequence of such failure and is therefore divinely sanctioned, i.e. AIDS is God's wrath.

Obviously such a view has homosexuals particularly in mind (despite the fact that AIDS/ARC is not a homosexual disease) and draws much of its inspiration from the prophetic literature of denunciation in the Old Testament. To this extent, AIDS is understood as the prophetic sign and instrument through which God punishes transgressions and affirms the existing moral concensus. It is usually the latter which is the principal intent of such a response, showing itself to be essentially concerned with maintaining the status quo rather than reaching out to those in need. It is for this reason that it remains naive and uncritical about its own position, frequently choosing the rhetoric of scripture rather than into theological questioning. Such a response appropriates to itself alone the language of prophetic consolation[5] inspired by the compassion of God, His faithful love and enduring choice of 'sinful' Israel. Only those within the chosen group become eligible for the benefits of such an election while God's free and sovereign grace is made conditional on the conventions of a middle-class puritianism. There is a deliberate decision to ignore the prophetic challenge to the status quo in the championing of the poor, the outcast and oppressed.[6] Such a response knows little of the radical questioning of the justice of God and the facile assumption of a causal link between sin and suffering represented in the figure of Job. It has yet to discover the great prophetic and priestly function of intercession on behalf of those who are afflicted and abandoned within the community and also those without.[7] Surely any community which lays claim to the prophetic tradition, and presumes to speak on God's behalf, has to lay claim to the *whole* of the tradition if its prophecy is to be authentic?

However, there is also another dimension to this response. In maintaining that AIDS is God's punishment, there is not only a proposition about the nature of Divine approval and disapproval; there is also a proposition about the nature of God Himself. If we accept the implications of the fundamentalist response, then we are bound to speak not only of a God who hates sin but also a God who hates homosexuals, I.V. Drug users, infected children and haemophiliacs. Given that there are also many who sin in amassing wealth or in their use of power while continuing to remain in very good health, we are confronted with a God whose capriciousness masquerades as justice — a God who can offer no cure, but who clearly shares the same views about the nature of right and wrong as those who speak in His name. Logically, such a position cannot stop at AIDS, but an illness, disease or suffering becomes God's punishment, and it would be necessary to maintain that degrees of affliction are in proportion to the gravity of the sin. In the face of our experience of innocent suffering which is so much part of our world, any attempt to work out the justice of this divine calculus must breakdown for it leaves us with a God who would reveal himself as ultimately immoral yet nevertheless powerful in sanctioning the particular conventions and opinions of a given group. The history of Christianity is a stark and salutary witness to the dangers of appropriating God in this way. It is a form of idolatry which remains a constant danger for all churches. Ultimately, such a position commits us to a god who generates, and is generated by, fear; one who is manipulating and manipulated. It is hard to see what would count as *salvation* with a god who only offers a theology of tyranny.

Through the language and the form is that of the Christian tradition, the God implicit in this way of responding cannot be the God of Christian revelation. This is a God who does not know His Son, what He has done, or the price which He has paid. It is a God who has forgotten the meaning of the Cross and Resurrection of Christ. The essential problem with fundamentalism, in any form, is its failure to deal with the freedom of God and therefore the unconditional nature of His Love:

> For God so loved the world that he gave his only Son, that whoever believes in Him should not perish but have eternal life. For God sent the Son into the world not to condemn the world, but that the world be saved through Him.
>
> Jn. 3:16:17

If the response of fundamentalist Christianity is inadequate not only in its failure to offer a basis for ministry but also in its theological assumptions, there is another question which informs the frequently reserved or cautious response given by bishops and priests.

In its teaching the Catholic Church is unequivocal in its position that though a homosexual orientation is in itself not sinful, its sexual expression is sinful.[8] This teaching is more nuanced in its pastoral application, but it gives rise to a nagging dilemma which colours the Church's response: in ministering to those with AIDS or ARC, is the Church implicitly condoning homosexual activity? It is not always easy to gauge the seriousness of the question in the face of the human need. If the answer is affirmative, would that justify no ministry to persons with AIDS or ARC, on the grounds of maintaining doctrinal coherence and pastoral integrity?

It may be that it was just such a concern that inspired the priest and the Levite in the parable of the good Samaritan. It could well have been a different story if the Samaritan had first interrogated the injured and abandoned victim about his lifestyle before deciding to help him. Once again, the question perceives AIDS and ARC as essentially a 'gay' disease, and moral disapproval is allowed to dictate the limits of compassion.

Undoubtedly, at the moment, the largest proportion of people with AIDS or ARC are gay, and many are in committed, permanent relationships. The Bishops conferences, both in America and Europe, have already addressed the situation and indicated their guidelines for a pastoral ministry which is consonant with the Catholic tradition.[9] Pastoral practice is also long used to distinguishing between acceptance and approval, as it tries to reach out to all who are seeking to live and practise their faith as well as those who need to know the overwhelming love of Christ and whose situation gives them a special claim upon it. The pastoral care which all the people of God claim of their pastors and Bishops by right of their baptism must not only nourish and deepen the union between the person and the community of faith through living a life 'worthy of the gospel', but it must also recognise and acknowledge the grace that is so clearly evident in many lives and situations.

At the pastoral level of the Church's life, the situation is often that of the parable in Mathew 13:24–30. The Church is subject to the discipline of reality with all its complex ambiguities and fragile histories, knowing that in these, too, there is the encounter with God's graciousness and human goodness. It requires a recognition that many things must wait upon God and His time. The pastoral ministry is truly a work of faith and trust and always one that, of necessity, must be open to the Spirit who accomplishes all things according to their seasons and who alone governs the 'kairos' of our lives and history. It must therefore be a ministry which has a deep and prayerful docility at the centre of its action; one which is not afraid to be surprised or challenged by the Lord and Giver of Life. If it lacks this, then it becomes either a safe ministry only to those who are safe, or an exercise in maintaining community discipline. Indeed, the situation begins to look very similar to those occasions in the gospels when Jesus finds himself in dispute with the pharisees: it becomes a question of what integrity means. Jesus' critique of their position is essentially twofold:

Firstly, the Law is the gift of God to the community. Its object is the celebration and sanctification at both the individual and communal level of the nation's relationship to the Creator. Yet the Creator is also 'Father', the one who has established the community, not just physically as He has with all creation, but also by His convenantal grace and love. The Law is, in its essential nature, the guarantor of this. However, to focus on the Law as an end in itself is ultimately to de-humanise it and empty it of its theological significance.
Secondly, the Law has been allowed to proscribe the range of God's actions so that He cannot act outside its boundaries. As the law instantiates the relationship between God and His people, but does not create it, so the Law is always subject to, and understood in, the freedom of God's Spirit to act where He chooses and to elect whom He will.[10] (The gospels themselves are particularly sensitive to this reality in their narratives of Jesus' birth).

It is always *God* who determines the boundaries of the community, because the community, as His creation, is not determined by the interpretation of the law at the hands of another. This is part of the insight which Paul will develop with such radical consequences for the future of the young Christian Church. Only within these perspectives is the true nature and effect of the law preserved.[11]

The Kingdom is the fulfillment of the Law by the restoration of its charismatic character. It may be that any ministry which is an attempt to bring the life of the Kingdom, its healing and its hope, will find itself in tension with other understandings of the Law. It may also be the case that it is precisely in such situations that the meaning and value of the Law is discovered. However, whatever the niceties of the debate, the ministry to those with AIDS and ARC is essentially a ministry to human beings not to homosexuals or I.V. drug users. It is a ministry which resists the prejudice and destructiveness that the easy categorising of humanity entails. All Christian ministry which engages the world is, of its very character, a ministry against any reduction or obliteration of the human face of Christ. It is a ministry of life over death, whether that death comes through economic deprivation, political oppression or a disease like AIDS or ARC.
In examining some of the questions which already have been part of the Christian community's response to people with AIDS or ARC, the dimensions of an authentic ministry

begin to emerge. It is one which has a genuine prophetic quality and content; one which is concerned with witnessing to the Kingdom. Such a ministry must cause us to reflect upon the boundaries of the community, the dynamic outreaching of God's love which constantly expands and challenges the limitations of our moral and political systems. It is a ministry which proceeds from the vision of faith, perceiving, behind the sophisticated arguments and the seemingly prudent manoeuvres about the provision and allocation of resources, a human face. This is true of all ministry, whether we are talking about the famine in Ethiopia, the situation in Nicaragua, or the poverty, despair and cry for help that we meet daily on our own streets. The Church's ministry to those with AIDS or ARC is part of the Church's fundamental option for the poor and marginalised; it is part of her mission against justice. It is nothing less than her option for Christ.

THE DYNAMIC FORM OF CHRISTIAN MINISTRY

There are many agencies and groups addressing the issue of AIDS and ARC to which the Christian community also feels itself called to respond. However, when the community understands its response in terms of *ministry* it is recognising:

1. It is not simply the work of a particular group or section but of the *whole* community. To this extent the whole community must recognise itself in the action and the form of the work.

2. Although always manifested in practical action which directly addresses the material and spiritual situation of those in need there is an inner dynamic and a theological understanding which must be present if a ministry is to be fully Christian.

The essence of this dynamic is the Incarnation, and therefore any genuine ministry has a deeply Christocentric focus: it is under the direction of the Spirit witnessing to the presence of the Risen Lord. This dynamic comes from the way in which the Spirit realises a dialectic which is both *of Christ* and *to Christ.*

THE MINISTRY 'OF CHRIST'

The ministry which is of Christ is one which deeply strives to be authentically His because it knows itself to be a participation in His work of redemption. Its asceticism of self-giving is inspired by nothing other than the freedom of this privileged co-operation. In so far as it is rooted in this, it is a profound work of service, one which is open to the world in all its forms setting no boundaries in its desire to reach all men and women. It knows that no one is a stranger to God's love. This is a ministry which moves between the mandatum of Holy Thursday (Jn. 13:1–20) and the kenosis of Good Friday (Phil. 2:1–11); it is a ministry which lives and witnesses to the paschal mystery of Salvation. As a ministry of service worked out in humility, it belongs to the priesthood of all the people of God and is their vocation and charism. It is a ministry which is prepared to move beyond respectability and preconceptions in the asceticism of Love's self-emptying. In this ministry, the community knows itself to belong to Christ bearing the character of His Spirit.

THE MINISTRY 'TO CHRIST'

At the height of his ministry Jesus asks his disciples 'Who do you say that I am?' (Mk. 8:29). It is the question which is heard anew in the life of every person who is suffering, oppressed or outcast. The question is asked every time we pass them by or bring our presuppositions to bear upon their life and situation; each time we venture to define another person's value and identity in terms of our own canons of acceptability. Not only in his own ministry to the marginalised but also in his identification with them. Christ has given them the unique power to stand in His place and ask of us, His disciples, that fundamental question: 'Who do you say that I am?'

The ministry which truly hears and recognises this Christ knows that the question cannot be answered except in terms of Peter's profession of faith. It equally knows, with Peter, our own brokenness which is why the deepest form of ministry is always that of the woman in the house of Simon the Pharisee. In the inner reality of her action, a profound metanoia transcending convention and traditional form, we see the necessary basis for all our ministry. Her action is not lost, for it finds itself transfigured and redeemed in the action of Christ on Holy Thursday where it is taken up and transformed into the mandatum of service. This is the action of faith which affirms and is open to the reality of the Incarnation.

If our affirmation is not to be docetic in its practice, then it must be *here*, precisely where humanity is most under threat, that Christ is to be found. It is here that we are called to know humanity, not only as created in the image of God, but redeemed in the image of His Son: an image especially resplendent in those whose humanity and dignity is denied and defaced whether by suffering or bureaucracy.

These are some of the elements in any ministry which wishes to understand itself as the work of the whole community. In encountering persons with AIDS or ARC, it will have many different features which draw upon the rich human, spiritual and sacramental resources of the Church. As these have been written about in other places, [12] it is not necessary to elaborate them here. However, in the light of our own reflections it might be useful to identify some special dimensions.

INCARNATIONAL

Whatever has been his or her situation before, a person faced with AIDS or ARC is one who begins to walk precariously under the shadow of death or in the valley of a slowly debilitating and disabling illness. It is a journey filled with many fears, not the least of which is the fear that one often travels alone. There are the ultimate questions to be faced about the past and the future, the value and meaning of relationships. There is the question 'Who do you say that I am?' which is asked of lovers, family, friends and society. It is a question about what it means to be a person.

In the incarnation of His Son, God has so radically and completely made our humanity a part of His reality, that all humanity itself becomes a sacrament. This is the central affirmation and power of the ministry of one person to another. It is a celebration of the mystery of our faith. It means that no one stands alone or is beyond the reach of grace or love. We are ministers of this incarnational grace through our own compassion, love and understanding. Each gesture of service, each moment of presence, every practical act, no matter how small or routine, is a statement of faith in the reality of Jesus Christ[13] and is solidarity with Him in a concrete way: 'ubi caritas et amor Deus ibi est.'

The Incarnation therefore moves us beyond a humanistic compassion. For the Christian Church, compassion is not a noble gesture or a utilitarian love of neighbour, but a living out of the life of God's Son whose image is in my neighbour.[14] It would be wrong to think of this as an entirely one-way process. It has the character of the meal at Emmaus where in the breaking of the bread of suffering, and in the consecration of the cup of a person's life, our eyes are opened and the Risen Lord is seen. It is here too that such a ministry is one of hope and life. Life cannot be measured by its length, fame or affluence; it can only be measured by the quality of its faith and love — the extent to which it becomes a life belonging to others — one which knows that it has a future and for whom death is not, nor can ever be, the final word about our humanity. To see that in such a life Christ is living and has chosen to live, is to know that this life is secure and that death is only a change from life to fulfillment:—

Across my floundering deck shone
A beacon, an eternal beam. Fleshfade, and mortal trash
Fall to the residuary worm; world's wildfire, leave but ash:
In a flash, at a trumpet crash
I am all at once what Christ is, since he was what I am, and
this jack, joke, poor potsherd, patch, matchwood, immortal diamond
Is immortal diamond.

G.M. Hopkins
That Nature is a Heraclitean Fire.

RECONCILIATION

If it is a ministry which participates in the dynamic of the Incarnation, it is also a ministry of Reconciliation — for God was in Christ reconciling the world to himself. Reconciliation is the many-faceted reality of God's love and grace. At its deepest level, it is a restoration, an 'at-one-ment' with God, realised in the reconciliation with one's self in the broken and unfulfilled quality of our life which we can never complete or bring to completion on our own. It is a ministry of reconciliation to families and loved ones — a ministry of healing to all the relationships of a person's life. It is especially a ministry of reconciliation to the community of faith, bringing peace, the special mark of grace, which comes through God's acceptance of us as we are, in the certain knowledge of what we will be. The heart of reconciliation is truth accepted in love.

ECCLESIAL

Throughout these reflections, there has been the recognition of the ecclesial nature of all ministry. The Church's ministry to those who have AIDS or ARC says that they do not journey alone — the Christian *community* walks with them, not in fear or despair but in love and in hope. It cannot offer anything of itself but the fact that it is there, in solidarity, is the assurance that God is also present.[15] It is a ministry which asserts that the person with AIDS or ARC has a place in the Church — indeed the Church cannot be the Church of Christ without them. This also means that the Church must be actively engaged in advocacy. Where people cannot defend or speak for themselves or where governments refuse to make adequate provision, shifting resources from other needy groups instead of meeting the needs of patients without endangering other necessary programmes then, in justice, the Christian community must speak.

It is in reaching out to those in need that the community learns something of its own nature. The Christian community is created and sustained by the Word made real and active through the Holy Spirit. It knows the the Word is no abstraction or philosophical invention but is the human and historical person of Jesus Christ. If the community is to be the Church and not a social or religious institution then it must listen for and seek or religious institution then it must listen for and seek that Word throughout history if it is to have life. In the events of Easter and Pentecost, the community knows that, although the Lord belongs to the community, he cannot be contained by it. In this truth the Church is not only established but constituted as a pilgrim. The journey of the community is with the Risen one and *in search of* Him, until all time and History is fulfilled in His parousia. This means that the Church cannot stand outside history but is constantly called to shape and sanctify it, and to do this as the service of Christ. Perhaps in this respect, the most powerful image of the Church is in the women who wait upon the Lord throughout his ministry, especially at his crucifixion, and are present at his resurrection. They are those who are attentive and faithful at the hour of greatest need; they know that He belongs to them, but that they cannot possess or confine Him.

When the Church reflects upon the parable of the Last Judgement in Matthew 25:31, it knows the price of its failure to recognise him. The parable not only illustrates what is at stake, but also gives the criterion for knowing where He is to be found: in all those who are abandoned and unrecognised. What is interesting is the ambiguity, the hiddenness, of Christ's presence: He is where he is least expected; outside the boundaries of the community whose own expectations and values act as a sort of blindness. The Church's action, therefore, is not just one in response to Christ's commands but also one which is born out of a searching for Him beyond the pale of what is conventional or safe — in the poor, the abandoned, the afflicted and all those who are in suffering or in need. It is the choice of credibility over respectability, and only in this choice can the community successfully define itself as the community of *Jesus* rejecting the temptation of Donatism.

These are some of the features of a ministry to those who have AIDS or ARC. Clearly such a ministry is not an option but a command for a Church which takes its own theology seriously. It is a ministry which is about transformation and transcendence. Transformation of prejudices, reservations, disfigurement and death into the occasion of grace, a moment in which Christ is present. Transcendence in the following and recognition of the face of Christ; a leaving behind of the limitations and the questions, reaching out to the God who is always greater, forever calling us beyond ourselves to Him. It is a ministry which lives the prayer of St Francis:

Lord, make me an instrument of your peace
Where there is hatred, let me sow love;
Where there is injury, pardon;
Where there is doubt, faith;
Where there is despair, hope;
Where there is darkness, light;
Where there is sadness; joy
O divine Master, grant that I may not so much seek

To be consoled, as to console,
To be understood, as to understand,
To be loved, as to love,
for it is in giving that we receive;
It is in pardoning that we are pardoned;
It is in dying that we are born to eternal life.

Footnotes:

1. Paul VI. Octogesima Adveniens no.4., cf. also Evangelii Nuntiandi.

The most recent figures indicate that for this country there were already 490 full clinical cases by the end of August 1986. The official estimates of those infected run to about 30,000–40,000 but there is a recognition in professional circles that these are underestimated. The more realistic figure is likely to be around 60,000 or over and this will continue to increase.

In America, the most recent figures indicate that there are 2,348 people with AIDS; 18,000 with ARC; 60,000 who test positive. National estimates for the next decade project that there could be as many as 2–3 million who will test positive.

3. At present, in America, there are over 5,000 children between 1 month-5 years who have AIDS.
4. cf. The statements of Gerry Farwell and other fundamentalist Christians. An example is the Southern Baptist Covention President, Charles Stanley, who declares that God created AIDS to 'indicate his displeasure' with homosexual lifestyles. cf. San Francisco Examiner 9.1.86.
5. Is. 40:1, 2; 49:8ff; 51:17–23; 65:17–20; Jer. 30:10, 11; 33:14ff; Mic. 7:18ff.
6. Amos 4:1; 5:24; 8:4–8; Micah 3:1ff; 6:8.
7. Is. 64:10–18; Jer. 14:7–9; Gen. 18: 22 & 23.
8. Declaration On Certain Questions Concerning Sexual Ethics.
   Sac. Cong. Doc. Fid. 1975
   Letter to the Bishops of the Catholic Church on the Pastoral Care of Homosexuals.
   Sac. Cong. Doc. Fid. 1986
9. cf. Principles To Guide Confessors in Questions of Homosexuality. (American Bishops, 1973).
   To Live in Christ Jesus. American Bishops 1976.
   An Introduction to the Pastoral Care of Homosexual People. Bishops of England and Wales 1981.
   cf. Homosexuality and the magisterium. Documents from the Vatican and the U.S. Bishops 1975–1985. ed. J. Gallagher.
10. Mk. 2:1–12; 2:23–28; 3:1–6; Lk. 14:1–6. Matt. 9:11–13; 8:5–13.
11. Matt. 5.1.ff.
12. cf. The Pastoral Section. AIDS/ARC Program Information and Pastoral Kit. Diocese of San Francisco.
13. Gaudium et Spes III.38.
14. Gaudium et Spes I.12.
15. A Message to the People of God. §2. Extraordinary Synod of Bishops. Rome 1985, also Evangelii Nuntiandi §15.

CHAPTER EIGHT

A MORALIST LOOKS AT AIDS[1]

Martin Linskill

Elsewhere in this collection are forceful contributions from people who have been coping with AIDS first-hand. In comparison with their experience, which urges and challenges us to feel and care just as deeply, the pontifications of moralists, dispassionate and abstract in form, are bound to seem irrelevant, presumptuous, and even shocking. Their balanced rejoinder will be that, though without the passion their work cannot begin, without a certain detachment and generality they cannot reliably proceed, towards their wholly practical and not at all theoretical end of informing and guiding choice: for their discipline of ethics, or the science of morality, is the attempt to think clearly about what moves us strongly so that we may do rightly. In view of the confusions, emotions and quandaries that AIDS has precipitated, there can be no doubt that in addressing AIDS the moralist will be properly employed.

AIDS would seem to be in the main correctly described as a fatal, sexually transmitted disease. Because it kills, and has spread spectacularly, it has kindled exceptional public alarm, intensive medical research and specialist nursing care, and comprehensive official programmes of education and prevention on the part of governments. Here are clear areas of vocational and institutional responsibility — the duty to relieve and obviate suffering, the general obligation to take all necessary action to promote the common good, in this case public health — but the moral implications are wider than these: for everyone whom the phenomenon of AIDS alarms, there is a clear area of personal responsibility, too.

Most directly, since (we are told) the disease is chiefly transmitted by sexual contact and by exchange of blood, and since it falls within our competence to choose whether we have such intimate relations with other people as these activities imply or not, and in what circumstances we use or refrain from them, then AIDS is not a capricious bolt of fortune but a condition whose incidence or containment we can do something about — if we find it sufficiently important to do so. In the light, that is, and under the pressure, of values we hold and claims we acknowledge, our private efforts and intentions can make a difference. AIDS is a moral issue; not, for instance, a mere scientific challenge.

Less immediately, AIDS is a moral issue in the more familiar sense of inviting general, often heated, opinions, verdicts, and prescriptions in the direction of people 'responsible' who are conceived of as not ourselves. The public importance of AIDS may require me to take up some position with respect to it; but much of what I may judge 'needs to be done' I am in fact recommending should be done by other people, whose perceptions, priorities, and values may be different from mine, and of whose circumstances and constraining conditions I can only judge at a distance. Thus, my direct attitude towards people actually suffering from AIDS may well be conditioned by my remoter identification of some whole class of people as its propagators and typical or only victims. Notoriously, AIDS has been so assigned in the West, as a disease proper to certain minority social groups of whom conventional morality already disapproves, viz. homosexuals and drug abusers: so that a practical moral response to AIDS becomes complicated by prior value judgements on homosexual relations in themselves, resort to drugs in itself, and criminal activity in furtherance of either.

The moralist must insist that, whatever moral conclusions we draw, the facts we appeal to must be facts, and their interpretations valid interpretations. If, for instance, we're wrong about homosexuality and AIDS (we would be), or have misdescribed such linkage as there is (it has been), then whole sections of our moral arsenal become irrelevant. Ignorance and prejudice are not promising determinants of a moral point of view.

In addition to these formal strictures on careful reasoning, the moralist will also have a substantive contribution to make concerning values. Faced by so unambiguous but containable a social evil as AIDS, we are not, he can point out, hopelessly adrift in seas of subjectivity; for in any appeal, for instance, that people should change their pattern of behaviour, there fall to be weighed, to be accepted or resisted, only a limited number of consideratons of public and private good, right, duty, or fitness which can be readily specified.

The Christian moralist brings to these issues not further analytic skills but a distinctive and positive commitment, based on a strong conviction that there are objective moral values which are not dependent on what we happen to want but rather express what God has made and is drawing us to be, and an equally strong conviction that for the Christian, responsible moral choice is a cooperative work of God's grace in us, and one which is wholly 'customised' or proportioned to our actual limited and partial capacities of the moment: which is to say that more is not demanded of us than we can practicably bear or rise to. This combination makes Christian moral theology at once peculiarly insistent on ideals and peculiarly tolerant of and compassionate towards particular cases.

With so much by way of preamble, we can proceed to identify the properly moral questions concerning AIDS as follows:

i Personally and pastorally, how should we behave towards the people who actually stand under the disease or nearest it?

ii Critically, what do we make of contemporary public responses to it, whether negative or positive?

iii Practically and specifically, once we have correctly focussed the problem, how do our principles comport with what we are to recommend? — within which fall

iv two dilemmas of an ecclesiastical kind, concerning prevention, and

v two concerning care which arise from professional practice; and

vi Finally and most obviously moralisingly, what is that overall vision of human good which both controls our estimate of AIDS and prompts our particular response to it; what, positively, is our message or recipe of hope, our word of encouragement? This office of exhortation or edification is one the Christian moralist cannot forgo, for the traditional realistic optimism and grace-attending practicableness of his discipline compel him to it.

The remainder of this paper will address these questions in order.

I

AIDS with its related conditions is, first of all and straight-forwardly, illness. These are disorders, from and in which people are suffering — debility, despair, and death for the patients themselves (typically young and with lots to live for); crisis and grief for their families and friends; stress for the health workers who care for them. These are manifestly not human goods but (however occasioned) calamities which make the people needy people, needing the neighbour (medical or not) who will tend, comfort, and relieve where that may be, or help to bear what may not be, with that ready and loving alongsideness from which all sickness to some degree but especially this one isolates and insulates the sufferer. To respond in this way, if and as we are able to be 'there', seems a plain duty of humanity — Christians will add, as created (our dignity is owed it at one another's hands), as redeemed (the example and precept of Christ; this is part of what God loved and died for), and as sanctified (a clear ministry of paraklesis in the Spirit).

This is not the 'heavy compassion' so characteristically scorned by Edward Norman[2], nor is it a partisaned reduction to an impersonal cause, nor is it the commuted shock-response to what in other areas of medicine has been called 'shroud-waving'[3] — the raising, by particularly piteous appeals, of vast sums of money for projects of sometimes uncertain or disproportionately small utility.

Unlike these, this humane response remains personal, and is not comfortably hypothetical: there will be a 'there', if we are sincere in accepting what the AIDS-carers tell us, and own the duty of keeping ourselves relevantly informed.

II

There clearly is room, though, for some such deputed and systematic social response, in addition to the adventitious, personal one, the work of mercy; and ethical questions attend it. That there should be such widespread sympathy for so distressing a condition is reassuring; that it should look for some practical expression is laudable; that medical research should fall within it is an obvious good: but we shall want to be sure that these resources are being proportionately best bestowed, both in relation to our overall deployment of energy on AIDS, and with respect to all the other areas of medicine that equally need our money. AIDS the killer is undoubtedly becoming a successful 'shroud-waver', a fashionable charity (cf. the Windsor jewels), yet since elective behaviour is so large a component the moralist cannot help favouring a moral above a technical solution, even where both cost money. Rather than spend millions on the perfect anti-sun cream, might it not make better sense to persuade people to prefer the shade, or to change their driving habits rather than build bigger and better casualty departments? And again, since there is as yet no cure for AIDS, why has AIDS a larger claim on funds and publicity than, say, cervical cancer, also a sexually transmitted disease but one which is curable and currently afflicts far more people?[4] Such considerations of course in no way invalidate AIDS research in principle: to work to relieve suffering, even by these less proximate means, and to circumvent and cure disease, are most proper objects of the medical art, and may fitly reflect the divine compassion. The question is simply one of proportion, and calculation of the best-yielding direction of effort given limited resources.

Other responses to AIDS we can more shortly deal with; their claims to moral legitimacy mostly founder simply on the facts. Exaggeration of the communicability of the disease (whence ostracism of sufferers — even by doctors[5] — and panic chalice-measures in churches) may combine with misassessment of the persons or pratices at risk to make people already resented and marginalised into scapegoats for ills whose real roots and agents lie elsewhere. As the Chinese community suspected in a Sydney smallpox outbreak last century had their houses burnt down, so today we read of 'shoot the queers', of draconian and intrusive measures to test and quarantine first sufferers, then immigrants, then practically everybody, and even (it is alleged) the reader's letter proposal deliberately to introduce AIDS as a way of reducing the criminal population.[6] Apart from the logical confusion of reprisal and remedy and the moral enormity of in any way furthering disease, none of the factual presuppositions here hold. These suggestions either wouldn't work, or wouldn't be necessary or leave the real problem untouched.

III

They do, however, help us move closer to that accurate assessment of the problem which must precede and will wholly condition any proffered solution. The duty of present care is insistent, and to work for a future cure a proper calling; in the remaining area of prevention, the facts suggest, as we affirmed at the outset, that (if not quite without qualification) the risk of AIDS is eliminable at a stroke by what people choose to do or not do with their own bodies — specifically about sexual intimacy, about conception (in the light of materno-foetal transmission[7] of the disease), and about sharing needles and syringes. If we want, therefore, to do anything about the future spread of AIDS (a simple moral question), then this availability of choice is the place to start. The real enemy is not homosexual relations or drug abuse but (within or outside these activities) careless promiscuity and blood-sharing through needles; and the real friend is not coercive legislation or preemptive scientific breakthrough but the persuadability of human hearts and minds.

Let us first check out that what the newspapers call the 'battle against AIDS' is indeed a good and even required thing. Given what on any normal appreciation of human good has already been called an unambiguous social evil, it seems only the fanatics will dissent: those who view with complacency this display of God's displeasure at homosexual lifestyles[8], the already ravaged sufferer who vows to take as many of his persecutors with him as he can, the sponsor of AIDS as crime control. These unamenable categories apart — and even the 'wrath of God' school ought to be interested in reclamation and conversion — we may take AIDS-containment as an uncontroversial goal and education as the primary means towards it, judging that once those who are at risk plainly know the consequences, for themselves and others, they will be swayed by moral or at least prudential arguments to act responsibly.

IV

It is at this point that the promised dilemmas for those with an exacting personal morality arise. To achieve the desirable end of containing AIDS let us suppose it minimally necessary only to limit our sexual partners and be prophylactic, and only to regulate our drug equipment and be hygienic: how far then may churches or any other invited or self-appointed captains of morality and guardians of public order, in most effective pursuit of this straightforward public good, seem to do a deal with the moral nonconformists, to the extent of seeming to condone activities of which on other (but here not functionally pertinent) grounds they disapprove? Specifically, can the good outcome of minimising AIDS-spread by the recommendation of condoms be balanced against either the intrinsic evil of the irregular sexual relations which are still compatible with this advice, or the scandal to faithful and unbeliever alike of tacitly condoning such behaviour; and similarly in the second case; may not endorsement of a programme which urges, say, free sterile needles for addicts actually encourage a practice (withal illegal) that ought to be condemned?

As to the first, the Churches are not obliged to support anything without making both their principles and their reasoning clear, especially when even at the basest level of expediency their traditional teaching on absolute chastity will deliver the goods so much surely, and could (and therefore should) be urged even in quarters not receptive to theology. A recent Anglican report[9] doesn't recommend condoms, on the very sufficient ground that they don't work, and thus is not condoning anything. Its practical recommendation of chastity is uncompromised, though it envisages that not all who need to hear it will heed it. More acutely, it is evident that if AIDS is a (pragmatic) argument for chastity, it is a chastity so defined as, unacceptably to some, not to exclude stable relationships between homosexuals. Here too, within the strict limits of the problems of AIDS, there are practical counsels for the sexually active which outrun traditional Christian presumptions but need neither weaken nor suppress them in any campaign. There will simply be the pastoral question, how much of such teaching, and what presentation of it, will achieve the end in the circles where it most needs to be achieved.

On the question of drugs, the same Anglican parliamentary submission[10] noted that if new needles were given only for old, i.e. only to those who already used them, then the policy would not (unacceptably) increase addiction but (as intended) would help to save lives.

As with advice to homosexuals, it would be an instance of furthering a good for and with those who are not, realistically and as at that time, within reach of the best. Since there are people so circumstanced, whom the consequences include and to whom compassion should as surely reach, give them (we say) a saving word, be it only a little one, rather than a stone.

The Church walks into both these dilemmas, as into others often before, because she is persuaded that pressing public good requires her, and residual prestige makes it worthwhile for her, to address her moral exhortations beyond her usual constituency and into (not particularly heedful) secular society — and with the usual result, that at the consequences of the latter's unsmitten indifference (there being no community of ideal) she cannot but scrupulously writhe. Some may indeed predict that, as with divorce reform and the Abortion Act so here, for the sake of avoiding one evil (inextricable misery, backstreet health hazards, and now a subculture-specific epidemic) the Church will have ended up merely facilitating another — conditional marriage and easy divorce, irresponsible pregnancy and easy termination, promiscuity, perversion, and a persistent devaluing of sex. The analogy, however, fails and the real issue is different. In those cases the moralists either failed to see, or misjudged the enormous volume of, what else the new powers would permit: but in the case of AIDS there, first of all, are no new powers, nor any incentive to start doing what all are saying is so perilous; the intention is not the ambulance one, that the inevitable should be made less distressing, but the preventive one, that people's behaviour should change; and the desired result has already begun to happen (in the well-informed gay community)[11] before the moralists have even cleared their throats.

The issue is not that wrong things should start happening within the scope of right reasons but that an acceptable right thing should gain ground for a disquietly wrong reason. Already dismissed from the field, we Christian ethicists, by those who, accurately targeting AIDS education at the highly sexually active heterosexuals, demand a message 'neither dogmatic nor moralistic'[12], we need not kid ourselves that there is much Christian morality behind such a very limited continence as 'I'm more careful about who I sleep with; I get to know them better first.'[13] Even in cases where the new habits are nearer traditional chastity than this but their real dynamic has still been fear of disease, does anything remain of a virtue so interested, instrumentalised, and expedient; or will not, rather, the whole value of an external adherence to prescribed acts (or abstinence) be vitiated by defective intention?

In some schemes of Christian ethics this would indeed be so, where the whole value lies in our conscious conforming out of loving obedience to the Lord's command because it is the Lord's command; but not in the traditional natural law understanding of Western, Roman Catholic and Anglican, moral theology. This view does not shrink from saying that, although right intention is of course to be looked for as well (there will be many gradations), sheer right action obviously serves our interest even in itself, because it is nature working as it should, the smooth functioning of what we were made for by a loving, gracious, and constant will. We are therefore not reprehensible, just sensible, in choosing what is right ('merely') because it does us good — it will, whether immediately and prudentially, or, as Christians would claim, at much deeper levels too. If, as scares like AIDS suggest, being chaste by choice is like being sober, viz. a refraining from gratuitous hazard to your own or anyone else's health, then you are (and rationally) meeting your specification as a human being more successfully by the sheer fact of your non-promiscuity and non-inebriety even if you are in this state for rather mean and selfish reasons (which may under grace change, and higher ones — of thanksgiving, of self-offering — dawn in time). Even if it is fear that 'tricks' us into a stable relationship with a single partner, we are at least then in the right place to recognise (from within) the natural importance of human bonding, which arguably is the real value in and of sexual relationships together, and the real rationale of traditional constraints on sexual behaviour.[14] Unchastity or promiscuity is an evil because it frustrates that deeper bonding, and we may fairly use the evidence of AIDS, as of cervical cancer or tubal infertility, as some indication how ill adapted to promiscuity the human body is.[15]

By right sponsoring intention, sufficient urgent occasion, and objectively right prescription, we therefore judge that the scruples fail. The Church need not demur at an economical and pragmatic campaign of prevention, and the allegedly counter-productive and immoral tendency of such a thing is not established. There do remain questions: What does the Church say to the homosexual who is not promiscuous; Can her word to the lusty heterosexual be anything other than policy? but before addressing these in the final section we must note the other two promised dilemmas, which are not at all theoretical and self-indulgent but are confronting or will be confronting practitioners in the field.

V

The contemporary phenomenon of AIDS puts particular pressure for medical professionals on two familiar principles of their ethic of care, confidentiality and nonmaleficence. Should the doctor, first, respect the confidentiality of the AIDS sufferer, actual or prospective, who does not want an intimate third party told? The duty to attend to him and treat him at all is not in question — the doctor could not, ethically, for instance refuse him care simply because he disapproved of the sort of voluntary activity which had produced the condition[16] — nor is what is questioned his absolute duty to benefit his patient; but it would not be perverse to rule that the patient's presumptive right to what may be termed negative confidentiality (=non-disclosure) is in this case forfeit, through his neglect of his own positive duty in that regard (=full confiding) towards the one who is indefeasibly owed it, his sexual partner (given the particular character of the disease); and that the doctor might meet both his absolute and his contingent obligations better not by confidentiality but by at least strongly urging that the patient make the disclosure, and possibly, if he persisted in refusing, by informing him that his duty as a physician would bid him tell the third party himself — i.e., do just so much as would avert the harm that keeping confidentiality would cause. He would be in possession of life-threatening or life-saving information, concerning which he would meet his obligations even if the patient indefensibly neglected his — no doubt through fears which it would equally be the doctor's care to show were groundless or inappropriate. Is this presumptuous moral blackmail? It at least tries to preserve confidentiality by frankly discussing its limits, rather than simply regarding normal moral privileges as suspended and breaking the confidence. A case with such tightly specifiable circumstances would have no tendency to weaken the confidentiality principle in general.[17]

At a later stage in any such story, the illness can be so horrible as to make likely, insistent, and pitiful, requests from many quarters for euthanasia. Christian ethics will not, however, think the traditional principles appealed to in this area insufficient: that a distinction is to be drawn, and may not be crossed, between relief of suffering with dignity even if this should shorten life, and directly intending to terminate life, which is always impermissible.

VI

Human life is too trust-laden and interwoven a mystery to be bestowed and disposed of just as even the subject and bearer of it pleases. The very recognition of these constraining trusts and interweavings is where morality begins, and to respond to them as given, and as a mystery, but one ordered to a glorious and humanly engageable end, is the distinctive claim and programme of theology. For the Christian moral theologian, therefore, such autonomy or self-determination can only ever counterpoint the essential relatedness and beholdenness which experience and revelation alike report as the truth of our humanity. As a positive value (the very condition of moral responsibility at all), it can only work with and not against our ordained and proper status, capacities, and aptitudes, which are all of them defined by and ordered towards society and the life of the blessed Trinity its hope. In the Spirit is indeed freedom, that cooperative venture on the ideal starting from where I am; it is otherwise perversity, and that not metaphysical but demonstrable, in its effects both on ourselves as agents and on the (unheeded) rights, interests, and welfare of others.

To have attested these limits to freedom, and a recovered sobriety over the consequences for these delicate networks of trust, may prove to have been the chief and hardest lesson of the AIDS phenomenon. Having blighted an entire intimate area of personal gratification from which disagreeable cares and consequences had been supposed banished, it may perhaps now quicken a new deeper reverence and wider responsibility, which, were their antecedents not so tragic, would be only good, and cause for joy. Some moralists have with great relish depicted the horrors of AIDS as the crash of the permissive society[18]; this moralist, without grudging them their meed of prophetic doom, would sooner greet signs of any disciplined and wiser one that should take its place. Some there are: the message of AIDS that homosexual promiscuity can now only be grossly antisocial has sufficiently impressed the relevant constituency for the signs to be that their patterns of behaviour have indeed altered; and if we were to see the same shift in practice amongst promiscuous heterosexuals we should want to greet that, too, as not just a victory of fear but a re-perception of sanity and a move nearer home.

So, from our Christian perspective, it must seem; but to say so is more likely to patronise than to edify the people there is need to address. One of the strengths of the natural law approach has always been that it facilitates genuinely plural moral dialogue, without contentious claims to revelation and using instead only the values that commend themselves to anyone's reason — i.e., roughly, enlightened self-interest: morality can be expected to pay, to be what works, is our proper fulfilment and flourishing, not an arbitrary or impossible burden. It has, however, the two contrasting weaknesses that it is over-ambitious in presuming that its goods and ideals can equally plainly be seen, judged, and hailed as such from all quarters (if they're really so obvious and inherent, how come we miss them?), and that it seriously underestimates the complexity of moral failure, in leaving out the darker hues of guilt and sin, of fall or deviation from chosen and loved loyalties which it is a mistake to suppose are absent from even an unreligious person's experience of either physical suffering or moral perplexity. In other words, to view this outlook in the present context as a response to people who stand nearest AIDS: here is not enough starting-point-relativity for those whose sexual orientation means that traditional teaching has gone dead; not enough compunction and challenge for the confident and self-willed; not enough good news for the broken, haunted, and hopeless. Too much pricing and weighing, not enough tarrying and compassion; too much law to define, too little gospel to save. A full response to AIDS has to be more than — the people for whom the Church must speak her saving words are looking for more than — the supplying of correct judgement for use from positions of control.

Through his philosophical interests the moralist is probably bound to gravitate towards prevention, is bound to emphasize most the things that the independent agent can deliberately initiate, or the firm norms and principles in the light of which he should choose; yet none of these activities, of thinking, planning, and reasoning, is what the title of this paper promised, viz. looking at AIDS: and the answer and complement to the incompleteness and unsatisfactoriness, the arbitrariness and remoteness of the ethicist's formal contribution is surely here, in the looking. Looking, we are stirred and claimed by the needy, and looking, there is stamped upon us how great is the need. This beholding is not only a rekindling of compassion; it can bid a reproportioning of effort. Care and cure for me resumed their duly awesome and exigent proportions through two recent and arresting pictures. One was a photograph of figures in solidarity at an AIDS remembrance rally a year ago[19]; the other was a simple map of the continent of Africa, with almost the whole of it hatched in showing the distribution of the disease.[20] Not a dilemma or problem here, but gaunt, despairing, yet defiant faces, and gestures, of touched people; and not a self-inflicted hazard of a limited and sophisticated subculture, but the object of urgent and overstretched medical attention for the helpless on a world scale. To look is to be shown at length things hidden, and by love, late or soon, to be wounded. Only so can the pastor care, or the preacher comfort — or the moralist counsel.

Ascension Day 1987

References

1. An early draft of this paper was read to my students at Westminster College, Oxford, and has benefited (no doubt, not enough) from their reception.

2. Edward Norman, Aids: a task for the churches *The Times* Mon Oct 13 1986
3. Kenneth Boyd, Brendan Callaghan SJ and Edward Shotter, Life Before Birth 1986 pp 119 ff

4. As urged by A Singer, letter to *The Times* Tu Feb 3 1987
5. Tony Smith, AIDS: a doctor's duty *British Medical Journal* 3 Jan 1987
   Raanan Gillon, Refusal to treat AIDS and HIV positive patients *British Medical Journal* 23 May 1987
6. M D Kirby, AIDS legislation — turning up the heat? *Journal of Medical Ethics* 12/4 1986
7. Board for Social Responsibility of the Church of England Evidence to the House of Commons Social Services Committee's Inquiry on AIDS December 1986 (hereafter BSR: Evidence) s 14
8. James Hanvey, AIDS and ARC: A Theological Reflection On The Church's Ministry (reprinted here p. 33) *The Month* December 1986
9. BSR: Evidence s 9
10. ibid. s 13
11. Caroline Bradbeer, HIV and sexual lifestyle *British Medical Journal* 3 Jan 1987
12. ibid.
13. Young woman interviewed in *The Times* Wed May 13 1987
14. Cf. Jack Dominian, AIDS and morality *The Tablet* 10 January 1987 (reprinted here, p. 49)
15. BSR: Evidence s 6
16. Raanan Gillon loc. cit.
17. Grant Gillett, AIDS and Confidentiality *Journal of Applied Philosophy* 4/1 1987
18. e.g. Sir Immanuel Jakobovits *The Times* Sat May 9 1987
19. Above Jeffrey Weeks' article, Love In A Cold Climate *Marxism Today* January 1987 (reprinted here, p 27)
20. In *Daystar*, journal of the Franciscan Missionary Sisters for Africa, Spring 1987

CHAPTER NINE

AIDS AND MORALITY

Jack Dominian

A psychiatrist warns against drawing the wrong moral conclusions from the AIDS epidemic. A truly Christian morality can rest only on love, not on fear.

I find AIDS all the more distressing because the Christian community is largely unprepared to offer a convincing response, in terms of sexual morality, to the challenge posed by this terrible disease. To advocate abstinence from sex before marriage and faithfulness within it is to proclaim the traditional Christian teaching. But the world of today no longer accepts this teaching as a given. A case has to be made for it. In my travels both at home and abroad I find a singular absence of such a convincing case. And yet the catastrophe of AIDS is challenging us urgently to present the Christian teaching in its most persuasive light.

During the last quarter of a century, there has been a marked alteration in sexual and marital behaviour without an equivalent Christian reassessment. Two thousand years of Christianity have attuned us to link sexuality primarily with one objective: procreation. This has led to a morality largely based on biology, centred on the fusion of sperm and ovum and the approriate conditions for bringing this about. The insufficiency of such an outlook has always been obvious but the biological underpinning of sexual morality was shattered, with huge social implications, when the separation of procreation and intercourse became easy and widespread. This happened in the early sixties and the consequences have been dramatic.

NON-PROCREATIVE

Increasingly, throughout the world today, most marital intercourse is non-procreative. Ninety-nine per cent of sexual activity within marriage is knowingly and deliberately non-procreative, whatever the means of birth control which are used. So Christianity is faced with a new situation which is likely to remain with us permanently.

Some people may say that I exaggerate the extent to which Christianity has linked sex and procreation. Surely, they may ask, other purposes of sexual intercourse have been admitted: especially indeed, the strengthening of the love between the couple. Sadly, however, this has yet to be fully explored and understood. Very little has been written about it. As far as the Roman Catholic Church is concerned, the advances of the second Vatican Council on the meaning of sexual intercourse within marriage have largely been ignored because of the heated debate over Humanae Vitae.

Christianity can learn from the world in its attitude to sexuality. The world has widely sanctioned the goodness of sexual activity. This Christianity can unequivocally accept. Now is the time for Christians to disclaim any negative view of sexual intercourse. They can proclaim loud and clear that it is one of the most precious gifts of the Creator, with a richness of meaning that goes far beyond the biological.

The world has also gone far to break the link between sex and biology through widespread birth regulation. This has been a source of considerable anxiety to the Christian community, particularly to the Roman Catholic Church. This is not the place to return to the contraception controversy. It is the place, however, to assert categorically that what has to be considered is men and women as persons, and the link between them, based on love, rather than biological functions.

Lastly, Christianity can learn from the significant advances which the world has made during the last quarter of a century in understanding the formation and preservation of human bonding. The importance of sex as a basis both for mutual attraction and for the subsequent maintenance of marriage is receiving increasing attention particularly in psychological circles. This personal dimension of human sexuality has to be the foundation of the emerging morality.

Christianity rightly considers the family of enormous significance. Yet families are founded on the man-woman relationship which precedes the arrival of children, is responsible for their care and nurture, and survives several decades after their departure. No equivalent effort has been made to understand and service this relationship. It has taken large-scale marital breakdown to make us realise how much spouses in their own right need help and support.

Despite appearances to the contrary, the intense natural power of sexuality is not primarily directed towards pleasure or procreation, but towards bond formation and thereafter the maintenance of the bond formed. In the second chapter of Genesis God affirms, "It is not right that man should be alone". At the heart of the mystery of creation is relationship, and a loving relationship between man and woman is fundamental. A Trinitarian faith that believes in the mystery of three divine persons in relationships of love should not find the revelation surprising.

Thus Christianity should have no problem in proclaiming sexuality to be that force which impels men and women towards the formation and maintenance of an exlusive relationship. In practice when a man and woman are attracted towards each other, the impulse is towards sexual intercourse to complete the bonding process. But there is need for clarity here. The desire to have sexual intercourse in order to become one is part of the process of personal bonding; its significance cannot be confined to physical orgasm. Premarital promiscuity distorts the meaning of sexual attraction. The man or woman who seeks bodily pleasure in the absence of personal encounter is dehumanising all that sexual attraction seeks to achieve and the body can rebel against such treatment through venereal infection or cancer or both.

What our society needs to restore is the proper place of courtship. This phase ensures that sexual attraction acts as a stimulus for deepening awareness of each other as persons.

Some may say that premarital cohabitation achieves precisely this. Certainly such living together on a basis which is mostly exclusive and faithful is not promiscuity and should not be placed in that category. It is nevertheless sexual intercourse outside marriage. Here some would argue that the issue is not sexual morality but the nomenclature of marriage. At one period in the history of the Church such exclusive, faithful and committed relationships sealed with sexual intercourse were considered to be valid marriages, and some sociologists today regard cohabitation as part of marriage. Nevertheless, the stability of marriage is so important that it should be given every support, and the greatest possible strength is conferred by a public declaration.

SUSTAINING THE BOND

Once a permanent bond called marriage is established, modern health care combined with social change has reduced the biological link between intercourse and procreation to a minimum. What needs to be expanded enormously is our understanding of the role of intercourse in maintaining the husband-wife relationship for the growth and nurture in love of the children. I have written extensively about this in The Tablet and elsewhere. The findings of psychology have proved beyond question the need for children to be brought up by parents whose marriages are secure. We are being made increasingly aware of the tremendous damage inflicted on families by an unstable or broken marriage.

Intercourse is primarily concerned with the formation and maintenance of human bonds. When such a bond exists, extramarital intercourse is a violation of that relationship of love and threatens it, as well as causing immense pain. As repeated surveys have shown, society may hesitate to condemn premarital intercourse, but has no such reservation in condemining adultery.

As always when Christian teaching is authentic, the advocacy of faithfulness and premarital chastity does not inhibit but proclaims and assists human integrity. AIDS has drawn our attention to the need to avoid promiscuity, but we have to go far more deeply into the implications. At its simplest level, promiscuity is the pursuit of sexual pleasure, and in considering the matter many go no further. All of us working in the field of human relationships know that there is much more to it than that.

The man or woman who pursues sexual contacts relentlessly is often a deeply hurt and wounded human being who is incapable of forming stable loving relationships. These vulnerable people have often had very disturbed childhoods. The current large-scale marital instability is producing a vicious circle, for in turn the wounded children of such marriages are the potential alcoholics, drug addicts, disordered personalities, young offenders and sexual deviants of the future. The AIDS crisis must make us look more deeply at the instability of family life in the West.

Christian awareness in the field of sexuality and marriage has greatly increased, but there is still need for much more study. Against a background of such neglect, sexual abuse and marital breakdown are taking a severe toll. The arrival of AIDS is a reminder of the need to give priority to finding new ways of proclaiming the truth about sexual conduct and safeguarding the family, the fundamental human unit. For this, we need thought, funding and research. I have made such pleas repeatedly over the last 25 years and I am extremely sad that the occasion of a fresh call should be the potential disaster of AIDS. If catastrophe is to be avoided and effective progress in sexual and marital matters to be made, an enormous effort is needed and I appeal to everyone to make it. The world is hungry for the message.

But we must avoid simplistic solutions. Faced with the crisis of AIDS it is urgent and imperative that a sexual and marital morality based not on fear but on personal love should be established in the Christian community. St John makes it clear that fear and love are incompatible. In proclaiming love Christianity must not only advocate discipline and self-control, but also search the hearts and minds of ordinary people for the contemporary meaning of sexuality and marriage. We need to take all that is best in our tradition and combine it with the most recent advances made by the psychological sciences in understanding human nature, so as to present it anew.

CHAPTER TEN

WHEN A FRIEND HAS AIDS

James Hanvey SJ

Especially through his life style and through his actions, Jesus revealed that love is present in the world in which we live — an effective love, a love that addresses itself to man and embraces everything that makes up his humanity. This love makes itself particularly noticed in contact with suffering, injustice and poverty — in contact with the whole historical "human condition", which invarious ways manifests man's limitation and frailty, both physical and moral.

Dives in Misericordia §3

THE PRELIMINARY QUESTION

'What is the person who has Aids looking for from the Church?' This seems like a good question, the sort that any concerned person might ask. I have heard it asked by many people who feel that their faith requires some personal response to the present Aids crises. Occasionally, it is asked by priests and religious. It is also asked by Bishops and administrators, often under pressure to produce statements and devise strategies, conscious that AIDS is yet another area of modern existence where life seems to outstrip and expose the limitations of our neat conceptual frameworks whether they are moral, political or theological. Originally, it was the question suggested as the basis for this article.

However, this is not the first question, there is one which must take priority which is: Are you really open to the answer?

If, as individuals or as a community, we have not heard this question or asked it of ourselves then we run the risk of a response which remains an exercise in public relations or the shallow pragmatism of a crisis management, lasting only as long as the media decides or public attention permits.

Are you really open to the answer? questions the basis on which we come to people with AIDS or ARC (Aids related complex). Without doubt we come with all the usual good intentions, thinking, in fact, that we have something to offer. This is not obvious: many agencies and groups both in this country and in America recognised the need long before the Christian community and are engaged in deeply committed, generous and compassionate service purely on the basis of the human need. They work freely and openly without any of the prejudices and the extraordinary complex manoeuvres that Churches and hierarchies feel they need to go through. Although it is clear that AIDS is not a 'gay' disease, in America and in Europe the majority of persons with AIDS or ARC are, at present, homosexual. It is hard to avoid the impression that the Catholic Church is at least, embarrassed by this; a reaction often compounded by the fact that AIDS inevitably raises questions about sexual mores and practices. There is also the sense that the Church finds it difficult to separate the suffering and the need of the person with AIDS from his or her previous lifestyle. Indeed, many who have the disease will already have experienced hostility and alienation from the Christian community.

There is also another question which is addressed to the Church or anyone with a desire to help: How committed are you to those who have this disease?

It is clear that there will be no sudden cure and in many forms Aids, with all its related problems, will be with our society for a long time to come. Will you be there in the long nights and routine days as people try to maintain life as well as face death? Will you still be there with their families and friends, still prepared to develop the necessary human, spiritual and material resources? When all the panic and the paranoia has died away and public attention has moved on to something else, will you still be with those who have AIDS or ARC?

DISPOSITION FOR AN ANSWER

We have evidence that there is a deep desire among Christians to say 'yes' to all of these questions; to set out on this strange modern road to Emmaus: the pradigm journey of all the Church's pastoral ministry. Yet the journey has its conditions:

The openness to learning
Unlike most journeys there is no determined destination. There is just the hope that something of the love of christ will appear along the way. It is a journey which cannot have the security of answers in advance and therefore all who make it, even the Church, must be ready to learn. Learning means that we must be prepared to listen and this is not always easy for a Church which is used to giving answers and is often under pressure from people to supply them.

The openness to listening
Listening is the first action of love for its focus is on the one in suffering and in need. It is also a listening for the way in which the Spirit is moving through a person's life and experience. As with any sickness, not least with AIDS, the real teachers are those who are ill and unless we are prepared to recognise this we have nothing to give but our own prejudices and our tired, safe clichés. The pre-requisite for all of this is humility which comes from freedom — the freedom to meet another person on his or her ground, to accept a situation in which there are contradictions, in which all the forms of 'ego', whether personal or ecclesiological, have to be left aside. It is a freedom from the tyranny of responsibility whether moral, social or political. In the end it is the freedom to set out in search of Christ allowing Him to choose the place where He will meet us. It is also the freedom of Christ in His crucifixion. If we are not prepared for that then we have no place in this work for we will only contribute to the hurt, the frustration and the alienation of those who have the disease; we will only be adding our own needs and narrow preoccupations to an agenda which is already too full.

The capacity for Conversion
How we can help, are we prepared for the answer: Conversion — a change of heart?

> Conversion is the most concrete expression of the working of love and of the presence of mercy in the human world. The true and proper meaning of mercy does not consist only in looking, however penetratingly, and compassionately, at moral, physical or material evil: mercy is manifested in its true and proper aspect when it restores to value, promotes and draws good from all the forms of evil existing in the world and man.
>
> *Dives In Misericordia*
> *John Paul II (cf also # 4)*

Only if we are willing to allow the Spirit to work in us in this way by calling us beyond the security of our institutions and our categories to persons can we have something worthy to offer.

The first effect of this will be to change our question to not, 'what is a person looking for?' but, 'what do we do when a friend has AIDS?' When that is our question then maybe we will also have discovered the richness of our own life as Christian; may be we will have discovered here, with those we never saw or cared about before, the source of the Church's life: 'You are my friends' (Jn.15.14).

This is the reality and work of grace; God's free and unmerited gift of himself to us who also need healing. When a friend has AIDS all you can do, all you need to do, is love graciously.

> . . . it will be good to call attention to two points:
>
> 1: The first is that love ought to manifest itself in deeds rather than words.
>
> 2: The second is that love consists in a mutal sharing of goods, for example, the one who loves gives and shares with the one loved what he possesses, or something that he has or is able to give. . . . Thus one always gives to the other.
>
> Prelude to *The Contemplatio Ad Amorem*
> St Ignatius of Loyola. Sp. Exx. §231.

Aids is not a 'gay' disease, an 'African' disease or one that belongs to I.V.Drug users and to other minorities like children and haemophiliacs. It is a human disease and while all the moral, political theological and economic debates are gone at the centre, there are, and still will be, people. They are people of every class and type, some with many personal, social and spiritual resources others with very little. There are also the friends, the parents and the families with their questions, fears and needs as well. It is in this situation that the Christian community can offer its own rich resource of love and healing — it does have a ministry. It is the Spirit's imperative to walk with all those who are abandoned and alienated whether it is through suffering and debiliting illness or through moral, political, or economic oppression. (Gaudium et Spes §1.; Matt. 25.11ff.).

Although in many cases these people will find themselves on the fringes of the institution they are never on the fringes of the Church; indeed, they are at its heart.

Love has to be practical if it is to be real. AIDS and ARC like any fatal or debilitating illness robs us of ourselves. It is not just the physical humiliation or the anxiety, it is the need to know that we are still of worth and are still loveable. There is no unrealistic expectation of some sudden cure, there is simply the need for the really important things — friendship, company, humour and hope — the hope that you still matter to someone. Above all it is the need to know that you are not alone, that you can share all the questions, fears and anger as well as the grace and sometimes the fun.The first sacrament is the sacrament of our humanity and it is found in all the ordinary, routine things. It is found in the just being there through the long nights, in a touch, a smile or a kiss; it is found in the fact that even with AIDS and ARC life still goes on in all its mundane activity and not so divine comedy. When a friend has AIDS or ARC to be practical means that you first have to be there — the sacrament of presence. Anyone who loves can be its minister; no one is excluded from it and it is unconditional.

As in any situation which raises fundamental questions, it is not only the person who has AIDS or ARC who is challenged to reflect upon the meaning of his or her life and its values. Those who care for them, the Church and society, will also have to reflect. Often, caricatures and assumptions which are very deep seated will have to be left behind. There will often be a confrontation with our own prejudices and phobias, the instincts for survival and the search for scapegoats. It is also the time to rediscover values which we may have forgotten or the power in virtues which social fashions and theories had claimed were obsolete. The articulate prophets of sexual liberalism may well have proved false. AIDS and ARC present us again with an opportunity to think and to grow and perhaps reach a new understanding of and maturity in the things that matter. It may be offering us an opportunity to create a Church and a community in which people do not need to disguise or lie about what they as if they had been branded with some mark of Cain. It gives us the possibility of creating a Church in which people can live in the truth and with the truth, accepted and valued for their humanity. AIDS confronts us with our blindness and offers us all a time for healing. Really practical caring will not try to avoid these deeper and more radical dimensions by taking refuge in some sort of doctrine of 'moral neutrality' or benign pragmatism because such an approach is, in the end, also de-humanising and alienating.

Of course those who have AIDS and ARC also have their own prejudices and assumptions. There are those who have contracted AIDS through I.V. drug abuse and take some sort of moral refuge in the fact that 'at least I'm not queer'. There are some who will want to portray themselves as victims of a hostile society and those who find it difficult to accept responsibility for their own lives and actions. There are also many who have not the capacity for doing so even if they wanted. Whatever the circumstances, there is no one who does not need understanding and acceptance, if not approval.

Within this wide and complex spectrum there is perhaps one small group which calls for our attention: priests and religious who have AIDS or ARC. They are in a peculiarly isolated position. Given that the principal way in which

AIDS or ARC is transmitted is through sexual contact with an infected person the whole integrity and moral life of a priest or religious person is under scrutiny and exposed to public judgement. Often, for prudent and not necessarily punitive reasons, bishops and superiors have tried to avoid scandal and publicity. At times the way in which this has been handled has seemed lacking in compassion. A priest or religious person with AIDS or ARC is perhaps one of the most isolated and vulnerable members of the community. He will have deep and painful questions to face in the solitude of his own heart and conscience. Yet by vocation and calling he belongs to the community and the community cannot abandon him or pretend that he does not exist. As with all who are alienated and marginalised especially here the words of the prophets have power:

> For Zion was saying, 'Yahweh has abandoned me, the Lord has forgotten me' Does a woman forget her baby at the breast, or fail to cherish the son of her womb? Yet even if these forget, I will never forget you
>
> Is.49.14,15.

At the heart of priesthood is an austere and profound beauty. It is the sacrament of service which can only be realised through a deep self-emptying, a kenosis, in the name and image of Christ. It is for this reason that the sacrament belongs to the very being of the person. It becomes the form and horizon of his life and its meaning. As such it has an eternal reality before God and in the community of His people. It is never just a matter of function. Yet it is also lived in the changing patterns and circumstances of a human life. Even in frailty and brokenness a priest never loses his power to minister and indeed these very conditions of his life lead him in new ways of service. The Church should not be ashamed to recognise this.

When a person has AIDS or ARC he or she begins a long journey. If it is understood aright and accompanied by love it becomes a journey towards healing. The deepest level of this is reconcilation — reconcilation with the past and all the relationships and pain that have been part of the journey. It is also a reconcilation with the future, its fears of all the disfiguring and debilitating possibilities; the fear of losing control and dignity but most of all the fear of being alone and once more alienated. Even at the end, there can be the fear that God may hate you the way others seem to. How can you keep out the insidious and evil destructiveness of a moral and theological fundamentalism which dares to speak for a God it does not know? It is here, in this moment, that the Christian community knows the richness and the depth of the gift it has been given, for the source of its life is reconciliation. Out of its own knowledge and experience of the graciousness of the God 'who has reconciled us to Himself' it shares that gift with any one in need through all the different levels of healing — with God, with the past and the future of our own lives,, with friends and enemies, with all the experiences of our life and relationships. The community accomplishes this not only through its concrete sacraments but through its solidarity — its gathering of all those who stand alone in their pain and doubt and fear into itself. No one stands alone before God, they stand as part of a community which knows them and loves them, nourishes them and prays for them. Even at the moment of death the future is crowded with friends — there is always the Church that 'has gone before us marked with the sign of faith', a faith which is 'known to God alone'.

These are some of the dimensions and aspects of showing a practical and Christ-like love when a friend has AIDS or ARC. Clearly, their principle focus is on the personal and the way in which the Church is reflected in all the people who have AIDS and all engaged in this ministry. However, it would not be correct to conclude this reflection without drawing attention to another vitally important and practical action which the whole Christian community can do most effectively as precisely as a community.

Faith cannot be separated from the desire for justice. For the Christian, justice is not simply the requirements of law or a theory of political and economic structures, it is the work of Christ in His Cross and Ressurrection: justice is the work of reconciliation, the sign of the righteousness and mercy of God, a work of His love.

AIDS raises questions of justice and the Church

has a responsibility to speak out in the name of justice and compassion. It must speak out against the paranoia and all the phobias which threaten people's rights and would seek to deprive them of their basic dignity and privacy on the basis of an AIDS epidemic. Equally, it also has to remind individuals and groups in high-risk categories that the grace of belonging to a community also entails obligations. Those who have AIDS or ARC also have responsibilities — they also have to love practically.

In the allocation of resources we also have to be aware not only of needs but also of the requirements of justice. Money allocated for the care of patients and research into the disease should not endanger or restrict the funds available in other programmes for the vulnerable in our society e.g. the elderly, the chronically disabled etc. It may mean that once again we have to critically examine our priorities and the economic ideology which seems to be able to have contingency funds for military purposes but is unable to extend these to AIDS.

One of the most pressing needs for those who have AIDS or ARC is accommodation. Often when a person is diagnosed as HTLV positive they can come under pressure either from those they live with or landlords to move. They need 'safe' accommodation where they can carry on living as normally as possible without undue attention and harassment. At some point hospices will have a part to play but not every one wants to use them. As the number with AIDS increase and reach the terminal stage it is unlikely that they would be sufficent given the other demands upon them. It may be that hostels and day-centres provide a better option. The Christian community may find that it has the ability to help in making these resources available.

We also know that drug abuse is not the problem of the rich and famous. It is the young unemployed and homeless who are most at risk. If there is to be a real cure for AIDS or ARC then we also need to cure deprivation and expose the effects of the prevailing economic orthodoxies which generate and legitimise situations which leave people powerless and vunerable. We need to reexamine the sort of society they produce and assess their true cost to human beings.

So far the discussion and reflection of this article has been within the context of AIDS and ARC as a Western problem. We now know that it is not and that it threatens other countries which are much more vulnerable because they practically no resources to meet the demands that the disease makes. The obvious example is Africa. The most recent estimates indicate that as many as 2-3 million people may be carrying the virus and the majority are in their twenties and thirties — a crucial generation for the ecomonic and social development of emerging nations. When a friend has AIDS we must not only share ourselves and our expertise but our financial and material resources as well. The demands of friendship, justice and love are as universal as the Church. Africa is a friend.

CONCLUSION

When a friend has Aids there may not be much time to undertake a lengthy reflection of all the issues. There may not be much space even to ask many questions, we simply have to set out on the journey. Occasionally, on the way, we may glimpse the beginning of an answer, but perhaps most of all there may be a discovery that we can leave the questions and their demands for answers behind. In taking the risk to set out, to reach beyond our own doubts and boundaries, choosing to start with the mandatum of Holy Thursday — 'That you love one another as I have loved you' — even the Friday of AIDS and ARC must move forward to another morning with all its hope.

James Hanvey S.J.

APPENDIX A

IS IT SAFE? The Chalice and AIDS

THE CUP OF BLESSING . . .

Concern has been expressed about the possibility of catching AIDS from drinking from the same chalice as an infected person, during the reception of Holy Communion. This pamphlet has been produced to allay those fears and to look at the wider implications of such anxiety.

IT IS SAFE FOR ALL TO RECEIVE THE CHALICE . . .

The virus which is the cause of AIDS cannot be passed through the air or by using, for example, the same cups, glasses, door handles, towels or toilet seats.

The virus is very fragile and can only be transmitted directly into the blood stream. Surface contact is not sufficient to allow infection.

The wine used is, by its alcoholic nature, antiseptic and the chalice is a poor medium for transmitting any infection.

WHICH WE BLESS . . .

For any Christian to stay away from Communion for fear of AIDS or to feel unhappy about receiving Communion, greatly damages the symbolism of joining to Christ through his Body and Blood and with each other as parts of that Body. It helps to make the tragic sufferers from a terrible illness feel excluded from and unwanted by the Christian family of which they are a part.

IS IT NOT A SHARING IN THE BLOOD OF CHRIST?

We, as Christians, need to do four things:-

1. Remind ourselves and each other that we **all** need to drink deeply of Christ's compassion and forgiveness and to offer understanding to all our brothers and sisters as we gather to break the bread.
2. Reach out and touch all people affected by AIDS, realising that through the presence of Christ in all of us, we transform their suffering into a living example of God's love and compassion.
3. Correct the wounding misinterpretation of Christian teaching that AIDS is somehow God's punishment. God does not punish through suffering and disease.
4. Pray for those who have AIDS and those who have been exposed to the virus.

The Terrence Higgins Trust, the charity which informs and advises on AIDS, would be grateful for your prayers, your financial support and, if appropriate, your assistance as a volunteer.

— A PRAYER —

Loving God, you show yourself in those who are vulnerable,
and make your home with the poor and weak of this world;
warm our hearts with the fire of your Spirit.
Help us to accept the challenges of AIDS.

Protect the healthy, calm the frightened, give courage to those in pain, comfort the dying and give to the dead eternal life;
console the bereaved, strengthen those who care for the sick.

May we your people, using all our energy and imagination, and trusting in your steadfast love, be united with one another in conquering all disease and fear.

We make this prayer in the name of one who has borne all our wounds and whose Spirit strengthens and guides us now and forever.

APPENDIX B RESOURCE LIST

LEAFLETS

Aids: The Facts Aids: More Facts for Gay Men	Published by the Terrence Higgins Available free, send SAE.
The Facts about Aids — in conjunction with Thames Television Facts about Aids for Drug Users Aids: An issue for everyone Aids and HTLV III — A Medical Briefing Aids: To Test or not to Test An Introduction to the Trust	
Aids: Important new advice for Blood Donors	Available from the National Blood Transfusion Service.

ORGANISATIONS:

Terrence Higgins Trust	BM Aids, London WC1N 3XX. 01–833 2971
Haemophilia Society	PO Box 9, 16 Trinity St, London SE1. 01–407 1010
Health Education Council	78 New Oxford Street, London WC1. 01–637 0903
Gay Bereavement Project	Unitarian Rooms, Hoop Lane, London NW11 8BS
Christian Action on Aids	47 Venns Lane, Hereford. 0432–268167

BOOKS ABOUT AIDS AND HEALTH:

Aids: Questions and Answers	Dr V. G. Daniels, Cambridge Medical Books, £3.75
The Management of Aids Patients	Edited by D. Miller, J. Weber & J. Green, Macmillan, £10.95
Aids and the New Puritanism	Dennis Altman, Pluto Press, £4.95
Aids and the blood	Peter Jones, Haemophilia Society, £2.00
The Aids epidemic	Kevin Cahill, Hutchinson, £3.95
Sexually Transmitted Diseases	David Barlow, Oxford University Press, £1.95
The Sunday Times self help book	Gillie, Pryce and Robinson, Granada, £3.95
Aids Nursing Guidelines	Royal College of Nursing, 20 Cavendish Square, London W1M 0AB, £3.75

WHERE TO GET MEDICAL ADVICE

Although medical advice may be available from your own GP, not every surgery is equipped to do the necessary tests for Aids or other sexually transmitted diseases. The best place to go for specialised tests is a Sexually Transmitted Diseases clinic which is usually found at your local hospital, and where you can be advised in confidence.

THE TERRENCE HIGGINS TRUST

This Trust, named after the first person to die from Aids in Britain, offers the public a variety of services, ranging from telephone counselling to individual crisis support. The Trust works with those with Aids and those who have been exposed to the Aids virus.

The Terrence Higgins Trust BM Aids, London WC1N 3XX